INTERMEDIATE FETAL MONITORING COURSE

Student Materials

AWHONN
Fetal Heart
Monitoring PROGRAM

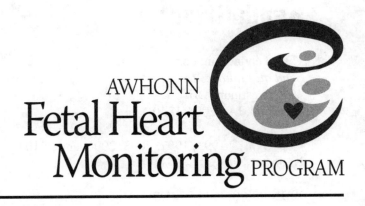

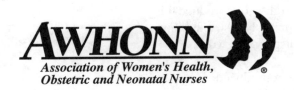

AWHONN
Association of Women's Health,
Obstetric and Neonatal Nurses

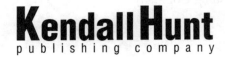

Kendall Hunt
publishing company

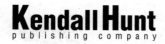

CONTENTS

INTRODUCTION AND SUPPLEMENTAL INFORMATION

Target Audience

The Intermediate Fetal Heart Monitoring Course is designed for healthcare professionals who have a minimum of six months clinical experience using fetal heart monitoring technology in the perinatal setting. It is expected that the participant already has basic knowledge and related skills in the following areas:

- Maternal physiologic changes of pregnancy
- Fetal growth and development
- Methods of fetal monitoring
- Preparation of patients for set-up and initiation of external or internal fetal monitoring
- Obtaining and maintaining tracings that document fetal heart rate and uterine contractions
- Interpretation of uterine contraction frequency, duration and baseline resting tone
- Identification of the baseline fetal heart rate, variability and variations
- Indicated clinical interventions
- Communication and documentation standards

This course is based on educational theory and the instructional design incorporates critical thinking and decision making. Residents, physicians, LPNs and LVNs may also participate in the course. To facilitate successful completion of the course, participants are expected, prior to attending the course, to review the current edition of the book *Fetal Heart Monitoring Principles and Practices*. Although the content of this course is comprehensive, specific patient care responsibilities vary according to institution, state, province or region. Those individuals who participate in this course are advised to be familiar with their organizational/institutional responsibilities, as well as competence criteria and measurement.

Acknowledgment of Commercial Support

This CNE/CME activity has been created without commercial support.

Sponsorship and Co-Providership Statements

The CNE activity is provided by the Association of Women's Health, Obstetric and Neonatal Nurses (AWHONN) in collaboration with co-provider, Professional Education Services Group (PESG).

This activity has been planned and implemented in accordance with the Essential Areas and policies of the Accreditation Council for Continuing Medical Education through the joint sponsorship of the Professional Education Services Group (PESG) and the Association of Women's Health, Obstetric and Neonatal Nurses (AWHONN). The Professional Education Services Group is accredited by the ACCME to provide continuing medical education for physicians.

Learning Objectives

At the conclusion of this continuing education activity, participants will:

- Analyze fetal heart rate patterns, uterine activity and their implications for fetal well-being.
- Discuss indicated clinical interventions and related maternal–fetal physiology.
- Effectively communicate verbal and written data about patient status.
- Describe the roles and responsibilities of healthcare providers in the use of FHM in intrapartum care.
- Demonstrate the psychomotor skills used in FHM.

Content Validation Statement

It is the policy of AWHONN and PESG to review and certify that the content contained in this CNE/CME activity is based on sound, scientific, evidence-based medicine. All recommendations involving clinical medicine in this CNE/CME activity are based on evidence that is accepted within the profession of medicine as adequate justification for their indications and contraindications in the care of patients. AWHONN and PESG further assert that all scientific research referred to, reported or used in this CNE/CME activity in support or justification of a patient care recommendation conforms to the generally accepted standards of experimental design, data collection and analysis. Moreover, AWHONN and PESG establish that the content contained herein conforms to the definition of CNE as defined by the American Nurses Credentialing Center (ANCC) and the definition of CME as defined by the Accreditation Council for Continuing Medical Education (ACCME).

Disclosure Statement

It is the policy of Professional Education Services Group and the Association of Women's Health, Obstetric and Neonatal Nurses that the faculty and program planners and developers disclose real or apparent conflicts of interest relating to the topics of this education activity and also disclose discussion of unlabeled/unapproved uses of drugs or devices during their presentations. Detailed disclosures will be made available during the live program.

Conflict of Interest Resolution Statement

When individuals in a position to control content have reported financial, professional or personal relationships with one or more commercial interests, AWHONN and PESG will resolve such conflicts to ensure that the presentation is free from commercial bias. The content of this presentation was vetted by the following mechanisms and modified as required to meet this standard:

- Content peer review by external topic expert
- Content validation by external topic expert and internal AWHONN and PESG clinical staff

Educational Peer Review Disclosure PESG reports the following:

- **George J. Vuturo, RPh, PhD**
  CME Director
  Dr. Vuturo has no relevant financial relationships to disclose.
- **Lawrence Devoe, MD**
  Dr. Devoe has no relevant financial relationships to disclose.
- **Anne Santa-Donato, RNC, MSN**
  Director of Childbearing and Newborn Programs, AWHONN
  Ms. Santa-Donato has no relevant financial relationships to disclose.
- **Carol Elaine Brown, RN, BC, MN**
  Nurse Program Development Specialist, AWHONN
  Ms. Brown has no relevant financial relationships to disclose.

Accreditation Information

Association of Women's Health, Obstetric and Neonatal Nurses is accredited as a provider of continuing nursing education by the American Nurses Credentialing Center's Commission on Accreditation.

AWHONN also holds a California BRN number: California CNE provider #CEP580.
Accredited status does not imply endorsement by the provider or ANCC of any
commercial products displayed or discussed in conjunction with an activity.

The maximum CNE credit that can be earned while attending the Intermediate Fetal Heart Monitoring Course is 18 AWHONN contact hours. Participants must attend the entire course and complete the feedback document in order to receive the CNE credit.

Accreditation Statement—Physicians

Professional Education Services Group is accredited by the Accreditation Council for Continuing Medical Education (ACCME) to provide continuing medical education for physicians.

Credit Designation Statement—Physicians

Professional Education Services Group designates this educational activity for a maximum of 15.25 *AMA PRA Category 1 Credits*™. Physicians should only claim credit within the extent of their participation in the activity.

DISCLAIMER

This course and all accompanying materials (publication) were developed by AWHONN in cooperation with PESG, as an educational resource for fetal heart monitoring. It presents general methods and techniques of practice that are currently acceptable, based on current research and used by recognized authorities. Proper care of individual patients may depend on many individual factors to be considered in clinical practice, as well as professional judgment in the techniques described herein. Clinical circumstances naturally vary, and professionals must use their own best judgment in accordance with the patients' needs and preferences, professional standards and institutional rules. Variations and innovations that are consistent with law, and that demonstrably improve the quality of patient care, should be encouraged.

AWHONN has sought to confirm the accuracy of the information presented herein and to describe generally accepted practices. However, AWHONN is not responsible for errors or omissions or for any consequences from application of the information in this resource and makes no warranty, expressed or implied, with respect to the contents of the publication. Competent clinical practice depends on a broad array of personal characteristics, training, judgment, professional skills and institutional processes. This publication is simply one of many information resources. This publication is not intended to replace ongoing evaluation of knowledge and skills in the clinical setting. Nor has it been designed for use in hiring, promotion or termination decisions or in resolving legal disputes or issues of liability.

AWHONN believes that drug selection and dosage set forth in this text are in accordance with current recommendations and practice at the time of publication. However, in view of ongoing research, changes in government regulations and the constant flow of information relating to drug therapy and drug reactions, the reader is urged to check other information available in other published sources for each drug for potential changes in indications, dosages and for added warnings and precautions. This is particularly important when the recommended agent is a new or infrequently employed drug. In addition, appropriate medication use may depend on unique factors such as individuals' health status, other medication use and other factors which the professional must consider in clinical practice.

RESOURCES AND REFERENCE MATERIALS

The information within this section is provided to assist in your preparation for participation in the AWHONN Intermediate Fetal Monitoring Course.

The references were utilized in preparing the course content and may serve as additional resources for you during your course participation and in your clinical practice.

BASELINE VARIABILITY

The numbers (1) through (4) included in the following cells correspond to the numbers encircled on the Visual Assessment of Variability Scale.

Amplitude of FHR Change	Former AWHONN Baseline LTV Description	NICHD Baseline Variability Description
(1) Undetectable from baseline	Decreased/minimal	Absent
(2) Visually detectable from baseline, ≤5 bpm	Decreased/minimal	Minimal
(3) 6–25 bpm	Average/within normal limits	Moderate
(4) >25 bpm	Marked/saltatory	Marked

Adapted from Electronic fetal heart monitoring: Research guidelines for interpretation, National Institutes of Child Health and Human Development Research Planning Workshop, 1997, *Journal of Obstetric, Gynecologic and Neonatal Nursing, 26*(6), 635–640. Copyright: AWHONN.

Note: The exact language in the 1997 NICHD paper regarding minimal variability is "greater than undetectable" and less than or equal to 5 bpm. AWHONN has chosen the equivalent term "visually detectable" to clearly differentiate the definition of minimal variability from the definition of "absent variability," avoid confusion for users new to the NICHD terminology and emphasize the visual determination of variability.

VISUAL ASSESSMENT OF VARIABILITY SCALE

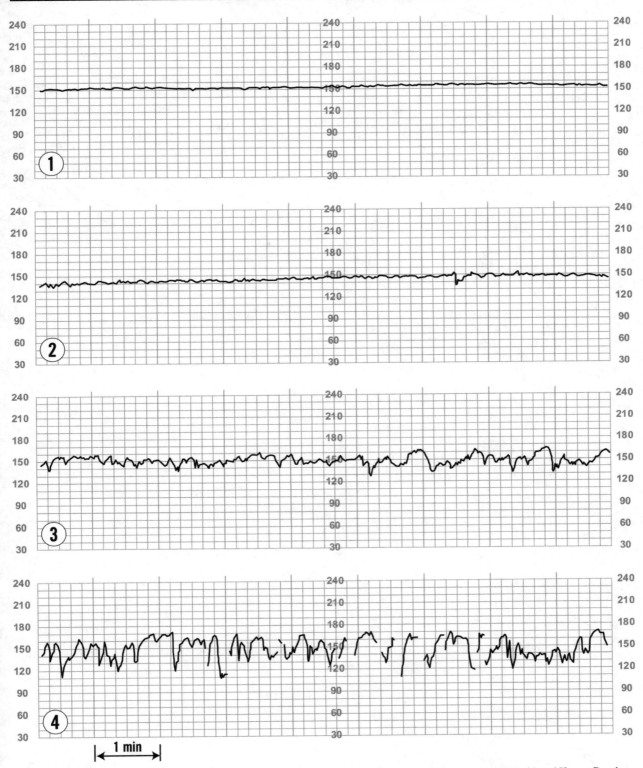

NICHD DESCRIPTIVE TERMS FOR FETAL HEART RATE CHARACTERISTICS

Term	Definition
Baseline Rate	Approximate mean FHR rounded to increments of 5 bpm during a 10-minute segment, excluding accelerations and decelerations and periods of marked variability. In any 10-minute window, the minimum baseline duration must be at least 2 minutes (not necessarily contiguous) or the baseline for that period is indeterminate. In this case, one may need to refer to the previous 10-minute segment for determination of the baseline.
Bradycardia	Baseline rate of <110 bpm.
Tachycardia	Baseline rate of >160 bpm.
Baseline Variability	Fluctuations in the baseline FHR are irregular in amplitude and frequency and are visually quantified as the amplitude of the peak to trough in bpm.
–Absent variability	Amplitude range undetectable.
–Minimal variability	Amplitude range visually detectable (>undetectable) but ≤5 bpm.
–Moderate variability	Amplitude range 6–25 bpm.
–Marked variability	Amplitude range >25 bpm.
Acceleration	Visually apparent ***abrupt*** increase (onset to peak is <30 seconds) in FHR above the adjacent baseline. The FHR peak is ≥15 bpm above the baseline and lasts ≥15 seconds but <2 minutes from the onset to return to baseline. Before 32 weeks of gestation, a peak ≥10 bpm above the baseline and duration of ≥10 seconds is an acceleration.
Prolonged Acceleration	Acceleration ≥2 minutes but <10 minutes duration.
Early Deceleration	Visually apparent, usually symmetrical ***gradual*** decrease (onset to nadir is ≥30 seconds) of the FHR and return to baseline associated with a uterine contraction. This decrease in FHR is calculated from the onset to the nadir of the deceleration. The nadir of deceleration occurs at the same time as the peak of the contraction. In most cases, the onset, nadir and recovery of the deceleration are coincident with the beginning, peak and ending of the contraction, respectively.

(continued)

Term	Definition
Late Deceleration	Visually apparent, usually symmetrical *gradual* decrease (onset to nadir is ≥30 seconds) of the FHR and return to baseline associated with a uterine contraction. This decrease is calculated from the onset to the nadir of the deceleration. It is delayed in timing, with the nadir of deceleration occurring after the peak of the contraction. In most cases, the onset, nadir and recovery of the deceleration occur after the onset, peak and ending of the contraction, respectively.
Variable Deceleration	Visually apparent *abrupt* decrease (onset to beginning of nadir is <30 seconds) in FHR below baseline. The decrease is calculated from the onset to the nadir of the deceleration. Decrease is ≥15 bpm, lasting ≥15 seconds but <2 minutes in duration. When variable decelerations are associated with uterine contractions, their onset, depth and duration vary with successive uterine contractions.
Prolonged Deceleration	Visually apparent decrease in FHR below baseline. Decrease is ≥15 bpm, lasting ≥2 minutes but <10 minutes from onset to return to baseline. A deceleration that lasts greater than or equal to 10 minutes is a baseline change.
Recurrent	Occurring with ≥50% of contractions in a 20-minute period.
Intermittent	Occurring with <50% of contractions in a 20-minute period.
Sinusoidal	Visually apparent undulating sine wave-like pattern in FHR baseline and cycle frequency of 3–5 per minute which persists for ≥20 minutes.

Macones, G. A., Hankins, G. D., Spong, C. Y., Hauth, J. D., & Moore, T. (2008). The 2008 National Institute of Child Health Human Development workshop report on electronic fetal monitoring: Update on definitions, interpretations, and research guidelines. *Obstetrics & Gynecology, 112,* 661–666; and *Journal of Obstetric, Gynecologic and Neonatal Nursing, 37,* 510–515.

REFERENCES

Introduction and Physiology

American Academy of Pediatrics & American College of Obstetricians and Gynecologists. (2007). *Guidelines for perinatal care* (6th ed.). Elk Grove Village, IL: Authors.

American College of Obstetricians & Gynecologists. (1999). *Antepartum fetal surveillance* (Practice Bulletin 9). Washington, DC: Author.

American College of Obstetricians & Gynecologists. (2002). *Diagnosis and management of preeclampsia and eclampsia* (Practice Bulletin 33). Washington, DC: Author.

American College of Obstetricians & Gynecologists. (2004). *Management of postterm pregnancy* (Practice Bulletin 55). Washington, DC: Author.

American College of Obstetricians & Gynecologists. (2005). Obesity in pregnancy (ACOG Committee Opinion 315). *Obstetrics & Gynecology, 106*, 671–675.

American College of Obstetricians & Gynecologists. (2007). *Screening for fetal chromosomal abnormalities* (Practice Bulletin 77). Washington, DC: Author.

American College of Obstetricians & Gynecologists. (2009). *Intrapartum fetal heart rate monitoring: Nomenclature, interpretation, and general management principles* (Practice Bulletin 106). Washington, DC: Author.

Catalano, P. M. (2007). Management of obesity in pregnancy. *Obstetrics & Gynecology, 109* (2 Pt 1), 419–433.

Gabbe, S. G., Niebyl, J. R., & Simpson, J. L. (Eds.). (2002). *Obstetrics: Normal and problem pregnancies* (4th ed.). New York: Churchill Livingstone.

The Institute of Medicine. (2003). *Health professions education: A bridge to quality.* Washington, DC: National Academies Press.

Joint Commission on Accreditation of Healthcare Organizations (The Joint Commission). (2004). *Preventing infant death during delivery* (Sentinel Event Alert No. 30). Retrieved December, 2009, from http://www.jointcommission.org/Sentinel Event Alert/sea_30.htm.

Larsen, L. G., Clausen, H. V., & Jonsson, L. (2002). Stereologic examination of placentas from mothers who smoke during pregnancy. *American Journal of Obstetrics & Gynecology, 186*, 531–537.

Lyndon, A., & Ali, L. U. (Eds). *Fetal heart monitoring: Principles and practices* (4th ed.). Dubuque, IA: Kendall Hunt Publishing.

Macones, G. A., Hankins, G. D., Spong, C. Y., Hauth, J. D., & Moore, T. (2008). The 2008 National Institute of Child Health and Human Development workshop report on electronic fetal monitoring: Update on definitions, interpretations, and research guidelines. *Obstetrics & Gynecology, 112*(3), 661–666; and *Journal of Obstetric, Gynecologic and Neonatal Nursing, 37*(5), 510–515.

National Institute of Child Health and Human Development Research Planning Workshop. (1997). Electronic fetal heart rate monitoring: Research guidelines for interpretation. *Journal of Obstetric, Gynecologic and Neonatal Nursing, 26*(6), 635–640 and *American Journal of Obstetrics and Gynecology, 177*(6), 1385–1390.

National Institutes of Health. (2000). Report of the National High Blood Pressure Education Program Working Group on High Blood Pressure in Pregnancy. *American Journal of Obstetrics and Gynecology, 183,* S1–S22.

National Institutes of Health, National Heart, Lung, and Blood Institute, National High Blood Pressure Education Program, NIH Publication No. 00-3029 (originally printed 1990, revised July 2000) and any subsequent updates. http://www.nhlbi.nih.gov/health/public/heart/hbp/hbp preg.htm. *The Journal of Clinical Hypertension, 3*(2) (p. 75–88). Abstract Full Test: HTML, PDF (1208K).

Parer, J. T. (1983). *Handbook of fetal heart rate monitoring.* Philadelphia: W.B. Saunders.

Parer, J. T. (1997). *Handbook of fetal heart rate monitoring* (2nd ed.). Philadelphia: W.B. Saunders.

Rasmussen, K. M., & Yatkine, A. L. (Eds.). (2009). *Weight gain during pregnancy: Reexamining the guidelines*. Washington, DC: The National Academies Press.

Smith, S. A., Hulsey, T., & Goodnight, W. (2008). Effects of obesity on pregnancy. *Journal of Obstetric, Gynecologic, & Neonatal Nursing, 37*, 176–184.

Interpretation

American College of Obstetricians & Gynecologists. (2003). *Dystocia and augmentation of labor* (Practice Bulletin 49). Washington, DC: Author.

American College of Obstetricians & Gynecologists. (2009a). *Induction of labor* (Practice Bulletin 107). Washington, DC: Author.

American College of Obstetricians & Gynecologists. (2009b). *Intrapartum fetal heart rate monitoring: Nomenclature, interpretation, and general management principles* (Practice Bulletin 106). Washington, DC: Author.

Bakker, P. C., Kurver, P. H., Kuik, D. J., & Van Geijn, H. P. (2007). Elevated uterine activity increases the risk of fetal acidosis at birth. *American Journal of Obstetrics & Gynecology, 196*, 313.e1–6.

Ball, R. H., & Parer, J. T. (1992). The physiologic mechanisms of variable decelerations. *American Journal of Obstetrics & Gynecology, 166*, 1683–1688.

Centers for Disease Control and Prevention. (2009). Births: Final data for 2006. *National Vital Statistics Reports, 57*(7). Retrieved December 14, 2009, from http://www.cdc.gov/nchs/data/nvsr/nvsr57/nvsr57_07.pdf.

Clark, S. L., Simpson, K. R., Knox, G. E., & Garite, T. E. (2009). Oxytocin: New perspectives on an old drug. *American Journal of Obstetrics & Gynecology, 200*, 35.e 1–35.e6.

Crane, J. M., & Young, D. C. (1998). Meta-analysis of low-dose versus high-dose oxytocin for labour induction. *Journal of the Society of Obstetricians & Gynaecologists of Canada, 20*, 1215–1223.

Daniel-Spiegel, E., Weiner, Z., Ben-Shlomo, I., & Shalev, E. (2004). For how long should oxytocin be continued during labor? *BJOG: An International Journal of Obstetrics and Gyneocology, 111*, 331–334.

Dare, M. R., Middleton, P., Crowther, C. A., Flenady, V., & Varatharaju, B. (2006). Planned early birth versus expectant management (waiting) for prelabour rupture of membranes at term (37 weeks or more). *Cochrane Database of Systematic Reviews 2006*(1), CD005302.

Feinstein, N. F., Sprague, A., & Trepanier, M. J. (2008). *Fetal heart rate auscultation* (2nd ed.). Washington, DC: Association of Women's Health, Obstetric and Neonatal Nurses.

Fox, M., Kilpatrick, S., King, T., & Parer, J. T. (2000). Fetal heart rate monitoring: Interpretation and collaborative management. *Journal of Nurse Midwifery and Women's Health, 45*, 498–507.

Freeman, R. K., Garite, T. J., & Nageotte, M. P. (1991). *Fetal heart rate monitoring* (2nd ed.). Baltimore: Williams & Wilkins.

Freeman, R. K., Garite, T. J., & Nageotte, M. P. (2003). *Fetal heart rate monitoring* (3rd ed.). Baltimore: Williams & Wilkins.

Garite, T. J., & Porreco, R. P. (2001). Evaluating fetal hypoxia with pulse oximetry. *Contemporary OB/GYN, 46*, 13–26.

Institute for Safe Medication Practices. (2007). *High-alert medications*. Huntingdon Valley, PA: Author.

Lee, C. Y., Di Loreto, P. C., & O'Lane, J. M. (1975). A study of fetal heart rate acceleration patterns. *Obstetrics and Gynecology, 45*, 142–146.

Low, J. A., Victory, R., & Derrick, E. J. (1999). Predictive value of electronic fetal monitoring for intrapartum fetal asphyxia with metabolic acidosis. *Obstetrics & Gynecology, 93,* 285–291.

Lyndon, A., & Ali, L. U. (Eds). (2009). *Fetal heart monitoring: Principles and practices* (4th ed.) Dubuque, IA: Kendall Hunt Publishing.

Macones, G. A., Hankins, G. D., Spong, C. Y., Hauth, J. D., & Moore, T. (2008). The 2008 National Institute of Child Health and Human Development workshop report on electronic fetal monitoring: Update on definitions, interpretations, and research guidelines. *Obstetrics & Gynecology, 112*, 661–666; and *Journal of Obstetric, Gynecologic and Neonatal Nursing, 37*, 510–515.

The Merriam-Webster Online Dictionary Retrieved December, 2009, from www.merriam-webster.com/help.

Parer, J. T. (1997). *Handbook of fetal heart rate monitoring* (2nd ed.) Philadelphia: W.B. Saunders.

Parer, J., King, T., Flanders, S., Fox, M., & Kilpatrick, S. (2006). Fetal acidemia and electronic fetal heart rate patterns: Is there evidence of an association? *Journal of Maternal, Fetal, and Neonatal Medicine, 19*, 289–294.

Parer, J., & Nageotte, M. (2004). Intrapartum fetal surveillance. In R. K. Creasy, R. Resnik, & J. D. Iams (Eds.), *Maternal–fetal medicine: Principles and practice* (5th ed.). Philadelphia: W.B. Saunders.

Phaneuf, S. Rodrigues Linares, B. TambyRaja, R. L., MacKenzie, I. Z. & Lopez Bernal A. L. (2000). Loss of myometrial oxytocin receptors during oxytocin-induced and oxytocin-augmented labour. *Journal of Reproduction and Fertility, 120*, 91–97.

Simpson, K. R. (2008). *Cervical ripening and induction and augmentation of labor* (Practice Monograph). Washington, DC: Association of Women's Health, Obstetric and Neonatal Nurses.

Simpson, K. R., & James, D. C. (2005). Efficacy of intrauterine resuscitation techniques in improving fetal oxygen status during labor. *Obstetrics & Gynecology, 105,* 1362–1368.

Simpson, K. R., & James, D. C. (2008). Effects of oxytocin-induced uterine hyperstimulation during labor on fetal oxygen status and fetal heart rate patterns. *American Journal of Obstetrics & Gynecology, 199*, 34.e1–5.

Simpson, K. R., & Knox, G. E. (2009). Oxytocin as a high-alert medication: Implications for patient safety. *Maternal Child Nursing, 34*, 8–15.

Society of Obstetricians and Gynaecologists of Canada. (2007). Fetal health surveillance: Antepartum and intrapartum consensus guideline. *Journal of Obstetrics and Gynaecology Canada, 29,* S1–S56.

Von Oech, R. (1983). *A whack on the side of the head.* Warner Books, Inc.

Williams, K. P., & Galerneau, F. (2003). Intrapartum fetal heart rate patterns in the prediction of neonatal acidemia. *American Journal of Obstetrics & Gynecology,* 188, 820–823.

Techniques

American Academy of Pediatrics & American College of Obstetricians and Gynecologists. (2007). *Guidelines for perinatal care* (6th ed.). Elk Grove Village, IL: Authors.

American College of Nurse-Midwives. (2007). *Intermittent auscultation for intrapartum fetal heart rate surveillance* (Clinical Bulletin 9). Silver Spring, MD: Author.

American College of Obstetricians & Gynecologists. (2003). *Dystocia and augmentation of labor* (Practice Bulletin 49). Washington, DC: Author.

American College of Obstetricians & Gynecologists. (2008). *Fetal lung maturity* (Practice Bulletin 97). Washington, DC: Author.

American College of Obstetricians & Gynecologists. (2009). *Intrapartum fetal heart rate monitoring: Nomenclature, interpretation, and general management principles* (Practice Bulletin 106). Washington DC: Author.

Declerq, E. A., Sakala, C., Corry, M., & Applebaum, S. (2006). *Listening to Mothers II on Childbirth Connection* web site, www.childbirthconnection.org

Feinstein, N. F., Sprague, A., & Trepanier, M. J. (2008). *Fetal heart rate auscultation* (2nd ed.). Washington, DC: Association of Women's Health, Obstetric and Neonatal Nurses.

Kleinman, C. S., Nehgme, R., & Copel, J. A. (2004). Cardiac arrhythmias in the human fetus: Diagnosis and therapy. In R. K. Creasy & R. Resnik (Eds.), *Maternal–fetal medicine* (5th ed., pp. 465–482). Philadelphia: W.B. Saunders.

Lyndon, A., & Ali, L. U. (Eds.). *Fetal heart monitoring: Principles and practices* (4th ed.). Dubuque, IA: Kendall Hunt Publishing.

Macones, G. A., Hankins, G. D., Spong, C. Y., Hauth, J. D., & Moore, T. (2008). The 2008 National Institute of Child Health and Human Development workshop report on electronic fetal monitoring: Update on definitions, interpretations, and research guidelines. *Obstetrics & Gynecology, 112*(3), 661–666; and *Journal of Obstetric, Gynecologic and Neonatal Nursing, 37*(5), 510–515.

Rouse, D. J., Owen, J., Savage, K. G., & Hauth, J. C. (2001). Active phase labor arrest: Revisiting the two hour minimum. *Obstetrics & Gynecology, 98,* 550–554.

Schwartz, N., & Young, B. K. (2006) Intrapartum fetal monitoring today. *Journal of Perinatal Medicine, 34,* 99–107.

Simpson, K. R. (2008). *Cervical ripening, induction and augmentation of labor* (Practice Monograph, Third Edition, Updated). Washington, DC: Association of Women's Health, Obstetric and Neonatal Nurses.

SOGC. (2007). Fetal health surveillance: Antepartum and intrapartum consensus guideline. *Journal of Obstetrics and Gynaecology Canada, 29*(9).

Choosing Physiologically Based Interventions

American Academy of Pediatrics & American College of Obstetricians and Gynecologists. (2007). *Guidelines for perinatal care* (6th ed.). Washington, DC: Authors.

American College of Nurse Midwives. (2002). The "push" for evidence: Management of the second stage. Washington, DC: Author. Press release retrieved December, 16, 2009, from www.midwifeinfo.com.

American College of Obstetricians & Gynecologists. (2006). *Amnioinfusion does not prevent meconium aspiration syndrome* (Committee Opinion 346). Washington, DC: Author.

American College of Obstetricians & Gynecologists. (2000). *Perinatal viral and parasitic infections* (Practice Bulletin 20). Washington, DC: Author.

American College of Obstetricians & Gynecologists. (2006). *Umbilical cord blood gas and acid–base analysis* (Committee Opinion 348). Washington, DC: Author.

American College of Obstetricians & Gynecologists. (2009). *Intrapartum fetal heart rate monitoring: Nomenclature, interpretation, and general management principles* (Practice Bulletin 106). Washington, DC: Author.

American College of Obstetricians & Gynecologists & American Academy of Pediatrics. (2003). *Neonatal encephalopathy and cerebral palsy: Defining the pathogenesis and pathophysiology.* Washington, DC: Author.

Andres, R. L., Saade, G., Gilstrap, L. C., Wilkins, I., Witlin, A., Zlatnik, F., & Hankins. G. V. (1999). Association between umbilical blood gas parameters and neonatal morbidity and death in neonates with pathologic fetal acidemia. *American Journal of Obstetrics and Gynecology, 181,* 867–871.

Association of Women's Health, Obstetric and Neonatal Nurses. (2008). *Evidence-based clinical practice guideline: Nursing management of the second stage of labor* (2nd ed.). Washington, DC: Author.

Barnett, M. M., & Humenick, S. S. (1982). Infant outcome in relation to second stage labor pushing method. *Birth, 9,* 221–9.

Chanraharan, E., & Arulkumaran, S. (2005). Acute tocolysis. *Current Opinion in Obstetrics & Gynecology, 17,* 151–156.

Fox, M. (2004). Obstetric emergencies. *Presented at Synergy: High Risk Obstetric & Neonatal Nursing,* November 4, 2004, San Francisco, CA.

Fraser, W. D., Hofmeyr, J., Lede, R., Faron, G., Alexander, S., Goffinet, F., et al. (2005). Amnioinfusion for the prevention of meconium aspiration syndrome. *New England Journal of Medicine, 353,* 909–917.

Gilstrap, L. C. (2004). Fetal acid–base balance. In R. K. Creasy, R. Resnick, & J. D. Iams (Eds.), *Maternal-fetal medicine: Principles and practice,* (5th ed., p. 434.)

Low, J. A., Lindsay, B. G., & Derrick, E. J. (1997). Threshold of metabolic acidosis associated with newborn complications. *American Journal of Obstetrics and Gynecology, 177,* 1391–1394.

Lyndon, A., & Ali, L. U. (Eds.). *Fetal heart monitoring: Principles and practices* (4th ed.). Dubuque, IA: Kendall Hunt Publishing.

Macones, G. A., Hankins, G. D., Spong, C. Y., Hauth, J. D., & Moore, T. (2008). The 2008 National Institute of Child Health and Human Development workshop report on electronic fetal monitoring: Update on definitions, interpretations, and research guidelines. *Obstetrics & Gynecology, 112,* 661–666; and *Journal of Obstetric, Gynecologic and Neonatal Nursing, 37,* 510–515.

Mead, P., Hager, W. D., & Faro, S. (Eds.). (1999). *Protocols for infectious diseases in obstetrics and gynecology* (2nd ed.). Oxford, UK: Blackwell Science Inc.

O'Grady, J. P., Parker, R. K., & Patel, S. S. (2000). Nitroglycerine for rapid tocolysis: Development of a protocol and a literature review. *Journal of Perinatology, 1,* 27–33.

Parer, J. T., King, T., Flanders, S., Fox, M., & Kilpatrick, S. J. (2006). Fetal acidemia and electronic fetal heart rate patterns: Is there evidence of an association? *Journal of Maternal–Fetal and Neonatal Medicine, 19,* 289–294.

Pullen K. et al. (2007). Randomized comparison of intravenous terbuataline vs. nitroglycerine for intrauterine resuscitation. *American Journal of Obstetrics and Gynecology, 197,* 414.e1–414.e6.

Roberts, J. (2002). The "push" for evidence: Management of the second stage. *Journal of Midwifery & Women's Health, 47,* 2–15.

Sarno, A., & Phelan, J. (1988). Intrauterine resuscitation of the fetus. *Contemporary OB/GYN, 31,* 143–152.

Simpson, K. R., & James, D. C. (2005a). Effects of immediate versus delayed pushing during second stage labor on fetal well-being. *Nursing Research, 54,* 140–157.

Simpson, K. R., & James, D. C. (2005b). Efficacy of intrauterine resuscitation techniques in improving fetal oxygen status during labor. *Obstetrics & Gynecology, 105,* 1362–1368.

Tucker, S. M. (2000). *Fetal monitoring and assessment* (4th ed.). St. Louis: Mosby.

Xu, H., Hofmeyr, J., Roy, C., & Fraser, W. D. (2007). Intrapartum amnioinfusion for meconium-stained amniotic fluid: A systematic review of randomised controlled trials. *BJOG: An International Journal of Obstetrics & Gynaecology, 114*(4), 383–390.

Communication and Accountability

Agency for Healthcare Research and Quality (AHRQ). (2006). *TeamSTEPPS: Team strategies and tools to enhance performance and patient safety.* Rockville, MD: Author. Retrieved December, 2009, from http://teamstepps.ahrq.gov/index.htm.

American College of Nurse Midwives. (March, 2007). Intermittent auscultation for intrapartum fetal heart rate surveillance (ACNM Clinical Bulletin number 9). *Journal of Midwifery and Women's Health, 52*(3), 314–319.

American College of Obstetricians and Gynecologists (2005). *Fetal heart monitoring.* (ACOG Practice Bulletin Number 70). Washington, D.C.: Author.

American Academy of Pediatrics & American College of Obstetricians and Gynecologists. (2007). *Guidelines for perinatal care* (6th ed.). Washington, DC: Authors.

American College of Obstetricians & Gynecologists. (2009). *Intrapartum fetal heart rate monitoring: Nomenclature, interpretation, and general management principles* (Practice Bulletin 106). Washington, DC: Author.

Association of Women's Health, Obstetrical and Neonatal Nursing. (2009). *Fetal Heart Monitoring* (Position Statement). Washington, DC: Author.

Chez, B. F. (1997). Electronic fetal monitoring: Then and now. *Journal of Perinatal and Neonatal Nursing, 10*(4), 1–4.

Clark, N. M., Cabana, M. D., Nan, B., Gong, Z. M., Slish, K. K., Birk, N. A., et al. (2008). The clinician–patient partnership paradigm: Outcomes associated with physician communication behavior. *Clinical Pediatrics, 47,* 49–57. Epub 2007 Sep 27. PubMed PMID: 17901215.

Feinstein, N. F., Sprague, A., & Trepanier, M. J. (2008). *Fetal heart rate auscultation* (2nd ed.). Washington, DC: Association of Women's Health, Obstetric and Neonatal Nurses.

Hickson, G. B., & Entman, S. S. (2008). Physician practice behavior and litigation risk: Evidence and opportunity. *Clinical Obstetrics & Gynecology, 51,* 688–699. Review. PubMed PMID: 18981793.

Hickson, G. B., Federspiel, C. F., Pichert, J. W., Miller, C. S., Gauld-Jaeger, J., & Bost, P. (2002). Patient complaints and malpractice risk. *The Journal of the American Medical Association, 287,* 2951–2957.

Joint Commission on Accreditation of Healthcare Organizations. (2004a). Focus on five: Strategies for enhancing physician-to-physician and staff-to-physician communication. *Joint Commission Perspectives on Patient Safety, 4*(11).

Joint Commission on Accreditation of Healthcare Organizations. (2004b). *Preventing infant death and injury during delivery* (Sentinel Event Alert 30). Oak Brook, IL: Author.

Joint Commission on Accreditation of Healthcare Organizations. (2005). 2006 critical access hospital and hospital national patient safety goals. Goal 2E "Implement a standardized approach to 'hand off' communications, including an opportunity to ask and respond to questions." Accessed August 8, 2005, at http://www.jci patientsafety.org/show.asp?durki=10293&site=164&return=10289.

Joint Commission on Accreditation of Healthcare Organizations. (2008). *Behaviors that undermine a culture of safety* (Sentinel Event Alert 40). Oakbrook Terrace, IL: Author.

Lyndon, A., & Ali, L. U. (Eds). (2009). *Fetal heart monitoring: Principles and practices* (4th ed.). Dubuque, IA: Kendall Hunt Publishing.

Preston, P. G. (2004). Presentation at Antepartum & Intrapartum Management Conference, June 19, 2004, San Francisco.

Royal College of Obstetricians and Gynecologists. (2001). *The use of electronic fetal monitoring* (Evidence-based clinical guidance number 8). London: RCOG Press.

Simpson, K. R. (2005). Perinatal patient safety: Handling handoffs safely. *MCN: The American Journal of Maternal–Child Nursing, 30,* 152.

Simpson, K. R., & Knox, G. E. (2003). Adverse perinatal outcomes: Recognizing, understanding and preventing common accidents. *AWHONN Lifelines, 7,* 224–235.

Simpson, K. R., & Knox, G. E. (2009). Communication of fetal heart monitoring information. In A. Lyndon & L. Ali (Eds.), *Fetal heart monitoring principles and practices,* (4th ed., pp. 177–210). Washington, DC: AWHONN/Kendall Hunt.

Society of Obstetricians and Gynaecologists of Canada (SOGC). (2007). Fetal health surveillance: Antepartum and intrapartum consensus guideline. *Journal of Obstetrics and Gynaecology Canada, 29* (9 Suppl.4), S1–S56.

Stelfox, H. T., Gandhi, T. K., Orav, E. J., & Gustafson, M. L. (2005). The relation of patient satisfaction with complaints against physicians and malpractice lawsuits. *American Journal of Medicine, 118,* 1126–1133. PubMed PMID: 16194644.

Evaluation and Synthesis

American Academy of Pediatrics & American College of Obstetricians and Gynecologists. (2007). *Guidelines for perinatal care* (6th ed.). Washington, DC: Authors.

American College of Obstetricians & Gynecologists. (2009). *Intrapartum fetal heart rate monitoring: Nomenclature, interpretation, and general management principles* (Practice Bulletin 106). Washington, DC: Author.

American Nurses Association. (2009). *Code for nurses with interpretive statements.* (2001). Retrieved December 17, 2009, from American Nurses Assocation.nursing world.org.

Lyndon, A., & Ali, L. U. (Eds.). (2009). *Fetal heart monitoring: Principles and practices* (4th ed.). Dubuque, IA: Kendall Hunt Publishing.

Macones, G. A., Hankins, G. D., Spong, C. Y., Hauth, J. D., & Moore, T. (2008). The 2008 National Institute of Child Health and Human Development workshop report on electronic fetal monitoring: Update on definitions, interpretations, and research guidelines. *Obstetrics & Gynecology, 112*(3), 661–666; and *Journal of Obstetric, Gynecologic and Neonatal Nursing, 37*(5), 510–515.

Membership Application

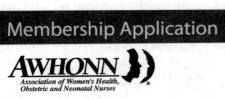

AWHONN
*Association of Women's Health,
Obstetric and Neonatal Nurses* ®

RECRUITED BY   (IF APPLICABLE):   RECRUITER'S MEMBER #:

MEMBERSHIP CATEGORIES (CHOOSE ONE)

☐ **Full $168**
RNs licensed in the
US, its territories or
Canada. May hold
elected and appointed
offices and may vote.

☐ **Non-RN $144**
LPNs, LVNs or others
interested in the health of
women and newborns.
May hold appointed office,
but may not vote.

☐ **Student $84**
Eligible for 4 years.
RNs may vote.
Proof of current
enrollment required.
Please attach.

☐ **Retired $84**
Must be at least 62 and
no longer working as a
nurse. Min. 3 years
previous full membership
required. RNs may vote.

☐ **International $192**
A nurse or other
interested party
residing outside
the US (other than
members of the
US Armed Forces).
RNs may vote.

PREFIX (MS, MR, ETC)   FIRST   MI   LAST   SUFFIX (JR., III, ETC)

CREDENTIALS (RN, CNM, ETC)   TITLE/POSITION (E.G. NURSE MANAGER, MIDWIFE, DIRECTOR, ETC)

HOME ADDRESS   CITY   STATE/PROVINCE

ZIP/POSTAL CODE   COUNTRY   HOME PHONE

EMPLOYER   WORK ADDRESS   CITY   STATE/PROVINCE   ZIP/POSTAL CODE

WORK PHONE   WORK FAX

PREFERRED E-MAIL ADDRESS FOR AWHONN COMMUNICATION

PREFERRED MAILING ADDRESS (CHECK ONE)   ☐ WORK   ☐ HOME

☐ I AM CURRENTLY AN ACTIVE DUTY MEMBER OF THE US ARMED FORCES. BRANCH OF SERVICE (CHECK ONE)   ☐ ARMY   ☐ NAVY   ☐ AIR FORCE
   (ACTIVE DUTY MEMBERS OF THE US ARMED FORCES WILL BE MEMBERS OF THE AWHONN ARMED FORCES SECTION.)
   RANK :

☐ I AM AFFILIATED WITH THE US ARMED FORCES (RETIRED, RESERVIST, DOD CIVILIAN, ETC) BUT AM NOT ON ACTIVE DUTY, AND I WOULD LIKE TO BE A MEMBER
   OF THE AWHONN ARMED FORCES SECTION INSTEAD OF THE SECTION IN WHICH I RESIDE.

WE OCCASIONALLY MAKE OUR MAILING LIST AVAILABLE TO CAREFULLY SCREENED ORGANIZATIONS THAT OFFER PRODUCTS AND/OR SERVICES THAT MAY BE OF
INTEREST TO YOU. ☐ CHECK THIS BOX ONLY IF YOU DO NOT WANT TO RECEIVE SUCH MAILINGS.

METHOD OF PAYMENT *

☐ CHECK OR MONEY ORDER PAYABLE TO AWHONN

☐ VISA   ☐ MASTERCARD   ☐ AMERICAN EXPRESS

CARD NO   EXP DATE

CARD HOLDER'S NAME

SIGNATURE

*DUES SUBJECT TO CHANGE. MEMERSHIP DUES ARE NOT REFUNDABLE.

AMOUNT ENCLOSED

DUES $

☐ OPTIONAL TAX-DEDUCTIBLE DONATION TO AWHONN   HEALTHFUNDS $30.00

TOTAL ENCLOSED $

ENTER PROMOTION CODE HERE, IF ANY

SUBMIT APPLICATION AND PAYMENT TO:
AWHONN, Dept. 4015, Washington, DC 20042-4015
Phone: 800-673-8499; 800-245-0231 (Canada)
Fax: 202-728-0575; www.awhonn.org

Member Profile

We want to make sure that we offer the professional nursing programs, services and products that are of greatest value to you. Please complete this member profile. Your answers will be kept confidential.

IN NURSING PRACTICE SINCE

_____

YEAR ONLY

DATE OF BIRTH _____

DAY MO YR

GENDER: ☐ M ☐ F

PRIMARY POSITION (SELECT NO MORE THAN 2)
☐ CASE MANAGER
☐ CLINICAL NURSE SPECIALIST
☐ CONSULTANT
☐ FACULTY-ACADEMIC
☐ NURSE EXECUTIVE
☐ NURSE MANAGER/COORDINATOR
☐ NURSE MIDWIFE
☐ NURSE PRACTITIONER
☐ RESEARCHER
☐ STAFF DEVELOPMENT
☐ STAFF NURSE
☐ STUDENT
☐ OTHER:

ETHNIC/RACIAL BACKGROUND (SELECT ONE)
☐ AMERICAN INDIAN/ALASKA NATIVE
☐ ASIAN OR PACIFIC ISLANDER
☐ AFRICAN AMERICAN (NON-HISPANIC)
☐ HISPANIC
☐ WHITE (NON-HISPANIC)
☐ MULTIRACIAL

CERTIFICATIONS (CHECK ALL THAT APPLY)
☐ AMBULATORY WOMEN'S HEALTH
☐ CHILDBIRTH EDUCATOR
☐ EFM/FHM
☐ HIGH-RISK OB NURSING
☐ INPATIENT OB
☐ LACTATION CONSULTANT/EDUCATOR
☐ LOW-RISK NEONATAL NURSING
☐ MATERNAL NEWBORN NURSING
☐ NICU NURSING
☐ NEONATAL NURSE PRACTITIONER
☐ NURSING ADMINISTRATION
☐ NURSE MIDWIFE
☐ OB/GYN PRACTITIONER
☐ PERINATAL NURSE PRACTITIONER
☐ PERINATAL NURSING
☐ WOMEN'S HEALTH NURSE PRACTIONER
☐ OTHER:

HIGHEST DEGREE EARNED
☐ DOCTORATE
☐ MASTER'S
☐ BACHELOR'S
☐ ASSOCIATE
☐ DIPLOMA
☐ VOC-TECH
☐ OTHER:

MEDICATIONS AND/OR OTC PRODUCTS (CHECK ALL THAT APPLY)
☐ HAVE PRESCRIPTIVE AUTHORITY
☐ RECOMMEND MEDICATION AND/OR OTC PRODUCTS
☐ COUNSEL AND EDUCATE PATIENTS REGARDING USE OF MEDICATIONS AND/OR OTC PRODUCTS
☐ NO ROLE REGARDING MEDICATIONS AND/OR OTC PRODUCTS

EQUIPMENT AND SUPPLIES (CHECK ALL THAT APPLY)
☐ MAKE PURCHASING DECISIONS DIRECTLY
☐ RECOMMEND OR INFLUENCE DECISIONS
☐ NO ROLE REGARDING PURCHASE OF EQUIPMENT AND/OR SUPPLIES

PRIMARY CLINICAL FOCUS (SELECT NO MORE THAN 2)
☐ ANTEPARTUM
☐ BREASTFEEDING/LACTATION
☐ INTRAPARTUM (INCLUDES LDR/LDRP & L&D)
☐ NICU
☐ NURSERY
☐ WOMEN'S HEALTH
☐ POSTPARTUM (INCLUDES MOTHER-BABY)
☐ OTHER: _____

JOB SETTING
☐ ACADEMIA
☐ AMBULATORY CARE (INCLUDES PHYSICIAN OFFICE, OUTPATIENT CLINIC, ETC.)
☐ HOME HEALTH CARE
☐ HOSPITAL INPATIENT
☐ NOT WORKING
☐ PUBLIC HEALTH
☐ SELF-EMPLOYED
☐ OTHER:

MAJORITY OF TIME SPENT (SELECT NO MORE THAN 2)
☐ ADMINISTRATION
☐ CONSULTING
☐ DIRECT PATIENT CARE
☐ MANAGEMENT/SUPERVISION
☐ PATIENT EDUCATION
☐ RESEARCH
☐ STAFF DEVELOPMENT/EDUCATION
☐ UNDERGRAD/GRADUATE NURSING EDUCATION
☐ OTHER: _____

IS CONTINUING EDUCATION (CE) REQUIRED FOR YOU TO MAINTAIN LICENSURE AND/OR CERTIFICATION?
☐ YES   ☐ NO

OTHER MEMBERSHIPS
☐ AACN (CRITICAL CARE NURSES) AANP ACNM ANA
☐ ANN AONE NANN NPWH SIGMA THETA TAU
☐ OTHER: _____

HOW DID YOU LEARN ABOUT AWHONN?
☐ COLLEAGUE
☐ ADVERTISEMENT
☐ MAILING
☐ CONFERENCE/CONVENTION
☐ OTHER: _____

SUBMIT APPLICATION AND PAYMENT TO:
AWHONN, Dept. 4015, Washington, DC 20042-4015
Phone: 800-673-8499; 800-245-0231 (Canada)
Fax: 202-728-0575; www.awhonn.org

COURSE OUTLINE

AWHONN Intermediate Fetal Heart Monitoring Course

© 2010 AWHONN 1

Course Objectives

- Analyze fetal heart rate patterns, uterine activity and the implications of each for fetal well-being.
- Discuss indicated clinical interventions and related maternal–fetal physiology.
- Effectively communicate verbal and written data about patient status.
- Describe the roles and responsibilities of healthcare providers in the use of FHM in intrapartum care.
- Demonstrate the psychomotor skills used in FHM.

© 2010 AWHONN 2

Disclosure

The Instructors of this course report either conflicts of interest or relevant financial relationships, or lack thereof.

The nurse planners for this course report no conflicts of interest.

© 2010 AWHONN 3

Disclosure (cont.)

The Instructors will discuss the off-label use of the medication terbutaline but will not be discussing the off-label use of any medical devices.

© 2010 AWHONN 4

AWHONN Fetal Monitoring Programs

- Clinicians' knowledge, experience and skills relating to FHM differ.
- The overarching goal of the AWHONN FHM Program is to provide a common foundation of knowledge and skills relating to FHM.
- Standardization of terminology for use by all clinicians promotes patient safety.

© 2010 AWHONN 5

2008 NICHD/ACOG EFM Workshop

- Revisited the report published in 1997
- Called the 2008 National Institute of Child Health and Human Development Workshop Report on Electronic Fetal Monitoring: Update on Definitions, Interpretation, and Research Guidelines
  - Provides definitions for categorization of EFM tracings

© 2010 AWHONN 6

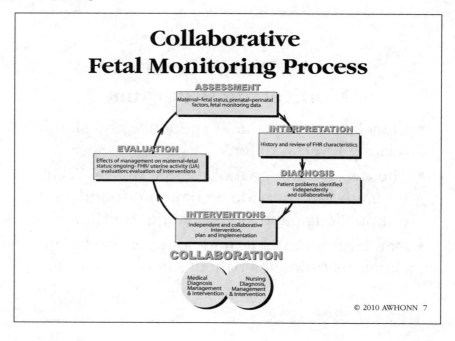

Collaborative
Fetal Monitoring Process

ASSESSMENT
Maternal–fetal status, prenatal–perinatal factors, fetal monitoring data

INTERPRETATION
History and review of FHR characteristics

EVALUATION
Effects of management on maternal–fetal status; ongoing- FHR/ uterine activity (UA) evaluation; evaluation of interventions

DIAGNOSIS
Patient problems identified independently and collaboratively

INTERVENTIONS
Independent and collaborative intervention, plan and implementation

COLLABORATION

Medical Diagnosis Management & Intervention

Nursing Diagnosis, Management & Intervention

© 2010 AWHONN 7

Assessment

Maternal and Fetal Database

© 2010 AWHONN 8

Assessment:
Maternal–Fetal Database

- History
- Family
- Medical/surgical
- Obstetric
- Psychosocial issues

- Current pregnancy:
  - Maternal assessment:
    - Medical/surgical history
    - Obstetric issues
    - Psychosocial issues
  - Fetal assessment:
    - Gestational age
    - Fetal activity
    - FHR

© 2010 AWHONN 9

Current Pregnancy

- Prenatal records:
  - Labs
  - Weight gain/loss
  - Vital sign trends
  - Ultrasound reports
  - Fundal height trends
- Patient interview

© 2010 AWHONN 10

Current Pregnancy (cont.)

- Physical assessment:
  - Maternal vital signs
  - Indicators of maternal–fetal oxygenation
  - Assessment of labor status (maternal)
  - Assessment of maternal and fetal tolerance of labor

© 2010 AWHONN 11

Cheryl, 35 Years Old
G_2, P_{1001}, 41 6/7 Weeks' Gestation

- History:
  - One spontaneous vaginal birth 8 years ago of a healthy 7 lbs, 4 oz (3,288 g) full-term male
- Family history:
  - Both parents hypertensive

© 2010 AWHONN 12

35 y/o ∴ AMA – offer amniocentesis

Cheryl (cont.)

- Current pregnancy:
  - First pregnancy with current partner
  - 10 prenatal visits
  - 47 lb (21.3 kg) weight gain
  - Fetal heart rate (FHR) and fetal movements within normal range throughout pregnancy

© 2010 AWHONN 13

Cheryl (cont.)

Estimated Gestational Age	Blood Pressure
11 weeks: first visit	120/76
20 weeks: second visit	126/86
26 weeks: fourth visit	124/84
35 weeks: sixth visit	140/88
37 weeks: eighth visit	136/86
40 weeks: tenth visit	130/88

BP trending up.

© 2010 AWHONN 14

Cheryl (cont.)

- 18-week Level II ultrasound confirmed dates by LMP and normal anatomy
- Fundal height exams consistent with EDC
- Quadruple screen
- Declined amniocentesis
- Second trimester glucose screen negative

© 2010 AWHONN 15

Cheryl (cont.)

- Admission:
  - 41 6/7 weeks' gestation admitted at 0500
  - Missed 41-week appointment
  - Vaginal exam: 2 cm/70%/-2
  - Fetus cephalic by Leopold's maneuvers and vaginal exam
  - Membranes intact, bloody show observed
  - Contractions: ① q 3–5 min × ② 40–50 sec; ③ moderate by palpation

© 2010 AWHONN 16

when assessing ctx use
* beginning to beginning of ctx OR peak to peak of ctx (NOT BOTH)

CTX- determine frequency q 3-5 min
                duration 40-50 sec
                palpation moderate

CTX — PERIODIC = occurs c̄ ctx
      NON PERIODIC = does not occur c̄ ctx

Cheryl (cont.)

- Admission (cont.):
  - Vital signs: BP 140/92, P 92, R 20, T 98°F (36.7°C)
  - Pain score 3/10
  - 3+ pretibial edema
  - 3+ patellar reflexes
  - Denies headache, blurred vision, scotoma and epigastric pain
  - Unable to void

© 2010 AWHONN 17

although pt is unable to void has signs i symptoms of PEC

Cheryl (cont.): Admission Tracing

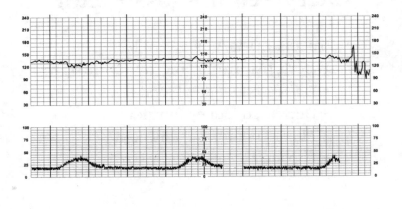

© 2010 AWHONN 18

Determine baseline c̄ one no. e.g. 135. not 130's - 140's /RANGE NORMAL = 110 - 160

Pertinent Historical Data: Hypertension (HTN)

Risks
- Maternal age
- First pregnancy with partner
- Family history of HTN

Signs and Symptoms
- Prenatal BP trends
- Weight gain
- Edema
- 3+ reflexes

© 2010 AWHONN 19

Cheryl (cont.): Risk Factors

- Preeclampsia/gestational hypertension/chronic hypertension:
  - Decreased uterine blood flow
  - Decreased kidney function
  - Altered neurologic function
  - Impaired liver function

© 2010 AWHONN 20

if PEC ⇒ ↓ blood flow ∴ ↓ uterine blood flow
↓ kidney function
altered neuro function
impaired liver function

Cheryl (cont.) Risk Factor

- Estimated gestational age: 41 6/7 weeks

© 2010 AWHONN 21

RISK FACTORS ARE INCREASED c̄ ↑GA

↑ GA

⇒ ↓ PLACENTAL FUNCTION I.e. calcifications, infarcts.

⇒ ↓ AMNIOTIC FLUID VOLUME

INFLUENCES ON FHR PATTERNS < EXTRINSIC = maternal

INTRINSIC = fetus

Extrinsic Influences on Fetal Heart Patterns

- Maternal affects blood exchange e.g. AMA, HTN, SMOKING, ASTHMA, DIABETES, SS DISEASE,
- Uteroplacental perfusion placenta & surface vessels.
- Umbilical circulation
- Amniotic fluid characteristics AFV maintained by Kidney function of fetus

© 2010 AWHONN 22

UTEROPLACENTAL PERFUSION can be affected by

- Late decels

- Variable decels

- prolonged decels

- change in variability (O_2 & CO_2 exchange affected)

Extrinsic Influences

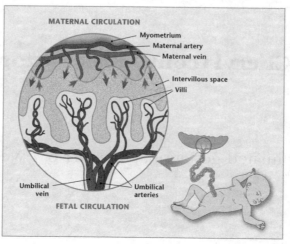

© 2010 AWHONN 23

Extrinsic Influences (cont.)

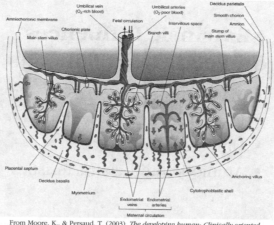

From Moore, K., & Persaud, T. (2003). *The developing human: Clinically oriented embryology* (7th ed.). Philadelphia: Saunders. With permission from Elsevier.

© 2010 AWHONN 24

Placental Aging: Calcification

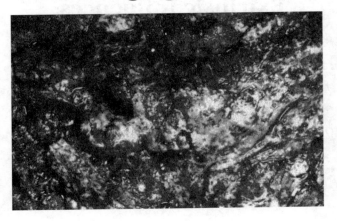

INFARCTION (yellow + white calcifications)

Placental Integrity Zone

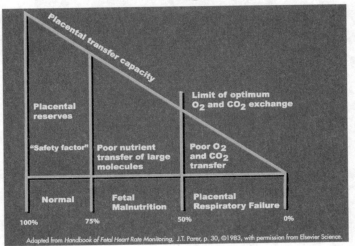

normal fetus has 2 times oxygen reserves needed

Extrinsic Influences: Placental Changes

- Hypertension:
  - Vasoconstriction
  - Infarcts
- Post-maturity:
  - Degenerative lesions (calcifications or infarcts)
  - Decreased amniotic fluid volume

© 2010 AWHONN 27

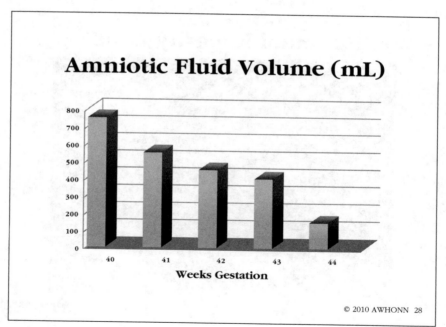

Amniotic Fluid Volume (mL)

Weeks Gestation

© 2010 AWHONN 28

AFV ↓ ↑↑↑↑ =7 losing cushioning effect of cord =7 ↓O₂/CO
=7 interruption of blood flow   exchang
4 fetus moves   =7 variable decel.
4 fetus does not move =7 prolonged decel
       if cord prolapse =7 bradycardia

. TEST - maintain maternal & fetal oxygenation by

Δ position
comfortable
proper O₂
↓ pain

Intrinsic Influences on the FHR:
Fetal Homeostatic Compensatory Mechanisms

- Fetal circulation
- Autonomic nervous system responses   FETAL
- Baroreceptors
- Chemoreceptors
- Hormonal responses

➡ Redistribution of blood flow to vital organs / SALVAGING
i.e brain, heart, adrenals

© 2010 AWHONN 29

INTRINSIC refers to fetus

CH. 2. FETAL CIRCULATION

Fetal Circulation

To brain
Ductus arteriosus
Left lung
Right lung
Left pulmonary artery
Foramen ovale
Left pulmonary vein
Ductus venosus
Liver
Aorta
Umbilical vein
Gut
Inferior vena cava
Umbilical cord
Umbilical arteries
Placenta

© 2010 AWHONN 30

° PRETERM FETUS
~ redistribution of blood flow
- NEC: due to
↓ blood supply to gut

fetus has twice the reserves that it needs during labor

if baro & chemoreceptors are not working well ⇒ change in variability

PRETERM FETUS
- have higher baseline because parasympathetic not mature.

A

TEST Q.
MODERATE FHR variability
- predicts absence of fetal metabolic acidosis

Regulation of Fetal Heart Rate and Blood Flow

- Cardioregulatory center/CRC
- Autonomic nervous system:
  - Parasympathetic - *slows down HR*
  - Sympathetic = *speedy*
- Baroreceptors - *↑ blood pressure Δ in aorta*
- Chemoreceptors ⇒ *↓HR*
- Hormonal responses

✓TEST Q. controls FHR baseline & variability
↓ maternal fever
↓ " pain ⇒ ta
k

(matures first)

↑ blood

✓TEST Q. vagus nerve stimulated then p
sym
cau
↓HR

Δ in O_2 & CO_2 ⇒ catecholamines release ⇒ vasoconstriction ⇒ ↑HR

↓ fetal BP ↓ sympathetic stimulated causing HR to ↑

©2010 AWHONN 31

MATERNAL FACTORS CAUSING SYMPATHETIC RESPONSE
- loud noise, ephedrine, atropine (anesthesia)

| BP ↓ | BAROReceptors stimulated Fetal pulse rate ↑ | ⇒ accels |
| BP ↑ | Fetal pulse rate ↓ | ⇒ decel |

SCALP STIM - assess parasympathetic & sympathetic recommended in absent variability

ANS / PARA SYMPATHETIC
     \ SYMPATHETIC

° PARASYMPATHETIC
- not mature in preterm fetus ∴ higher baseline
- medulla oblongata
- vagus nerve (10th cranial nerve)
- release ACH ⇒ ↓FHR

° SYMPATHETIC
- matures first
- nerve fibres in myocardium
- release catecholamines ⇒ ↑FHR

Intrinsic Influences on the FHR

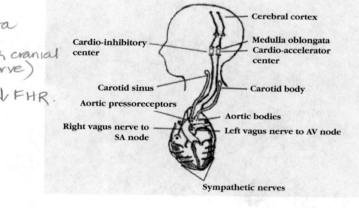

Cerebral cortex
Cardio-inhibitory center
Medulla oblongata Cardio-accelerator center
Carotid sinus
Carotid body
Aortic pressoreceptors
Aortic bodies
Right vagus nerve to SA node
Left vagus nerve to AV node
Sympathetic nerves

© 2010 AWHONN 32

° BARORECEP
- aortic arch carotid sin of ICA
- fetal arte
BP ↑ ⇒ va
nerve stimu
⇒ ↓ HR

° CHEMORECE
- regulate respiratory activities
- control c
- umbilica artery occ or hypoxemia ⇒ ↑ PCO_2 ⇒ stimulate che receptors ⇒
CRC ⇒ ↓FHR

Fetal Response to Stressors

Hypoxemia and/or decreased umbilical blood flow

⇩

Chemoreceptor/baroreceptor stimulation

⇩

Catecholamine production

⇩

↓ Blood flow to periphery (gastrointestinal and renal)

⇩

↑ Blood flow to vital organs (brain, heart and adrenal)

⇩

FHR changes
(Type of FHR change depends upon nature and timing of the stressor)

© 2010 AWHONN 33

If fetus has enough O₂ reserve it will compensate

Blood Redistribution during Fetal Hypoxemia

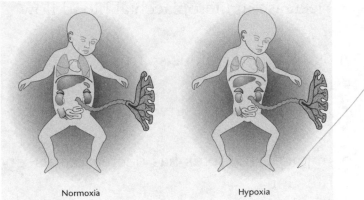

Normoxia   Hypoxia

© 2010 AWHONN 34

*IUGR FETUS
not proportionate*

*fetus c̄ large body
& small legs.*

*IUGR FETUR
↓ placental functioning
↓ AFV (⇒ loses cushioning)*

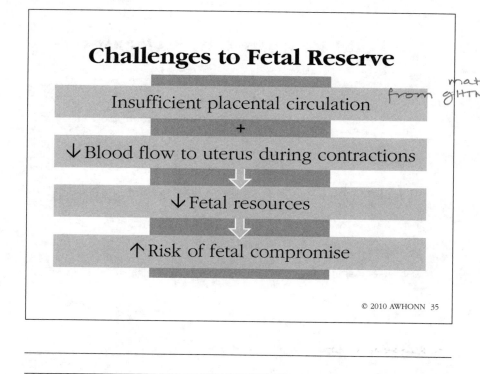

Challenges to Fetal Reserve

Insufficient placental circulation

from maternal gHTN, chronic H

+

↓ Blood flow to uterus during contractions

↓ Fetal resources

↑ Risk of fetal compromise

© 2010 AWHONN 35

Physiologic Stress of Contractions

- Decrease in uteroplacental blood flow

- Stasis in intervillous spaces

- Fetus relies on reserves

- Impact if the fetus has decreased placental function

© 2010 AWHONN 36

Fetal Reserve

- The degree of hypoxemia a fetus can tolerate before true tissue hypoxia and acidosis occur:

1. Placental transfer capacity *to transfer O_2*

2. Fetal homeostatic compensatory responses

© 2010 AWHONN 37

FETAL RESERVE
= safety net

COMPROMISED FETUS   htn => infarct in placenta
PRETERM FETUS   -   parasympathetic
                        less developed.

Fetal Well-Being

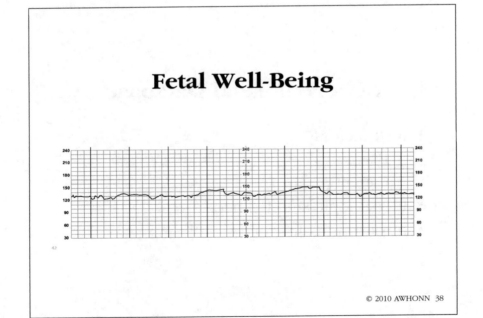

© 2010 AWHONN 38

TEST ✓
Q.

/MODERATE VARIABILITY ≥6-25 bpm
MINIMAL VARIABILITY ≤ 5 bpm
ABSENT VARIABILITY O = amplitude Δ undetectable
                        smooth, blunted, flat
MARKED VARIABILITY ≥25bpm

Dynamic Physiologic Response Model

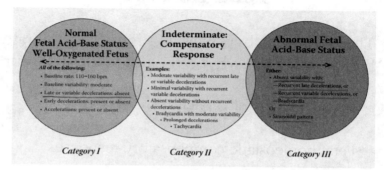

Fetal Heart Monitoring Principles and Practices, (2009). Association of Women's Health, Obstetrical and Neonatal Nurses. Used with permission.

© 2010 AWHONN 39

EARLY DECEL — normal due to descent of head
& compression.

Maternal–Fetal Database

- Risk factors:
  - History
  - Current pregnancy
- Physiologic significance
- Implications for fetal well-being

© 2010 AWHONN 40

Maternal and Fetal Physical Assessment

- Maternal vital signs and physical exam
- Fetal presentation
- Fetal movement
- Fetal heart assessment
- Uterine activity
- Labor progress

© 2010 AWHONN 41

INTRAPARTUM NOTE SHOULD INCLUDE THE FOLLOWING

Collaborative Fetal Monitoring Process

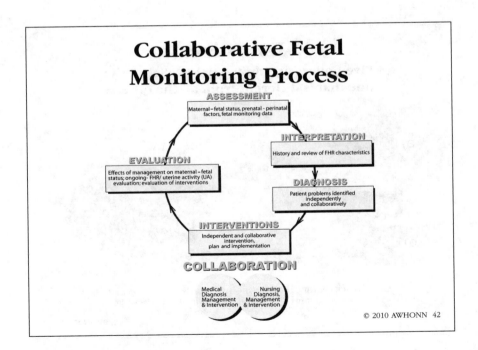

© 2010 AWHONN 42

Interpretation

Exercise

**Five figures are shown below. Select the
one that is different from all the others.**

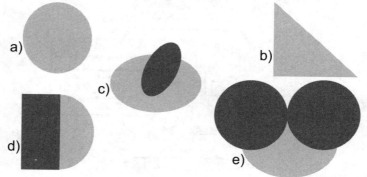

From A WHACK ON THE SIDE OF THE HEAD by Roger von Oech. Copyright 1983,
1990, 1998 by Roger von Oech. By permission of Grand Central Publishing.

Helga: Admission History

- Family medical history: unremarkable
- Medical history: allergy-related asthma   ↑ risk factors.
- Previous pregnancies:
  - Spontaneous abortion (SAB) at 6 weeks
  - 40-week spontaneous vaginal birth of 9 lb., 1 oz (4,110 g) girl   LGA = large for gestational age ↑risk factors
  - Postpartum depression for 2 weeks after birth => ↑ risk for depression

© 2010 AWHONN 45

DX: depression = 2 mths after birth

Helga: Admission History (cont.)

Current pregnancy:
- Routine prenatal care
- Prenatal labs within normal limits
- 29 lb. (13.2 kg) weight gain
- Admitted in active labor at 5 cm/80%/-1

© 2010 AWHONN 46

Helga (cont.):
Admission Tracing

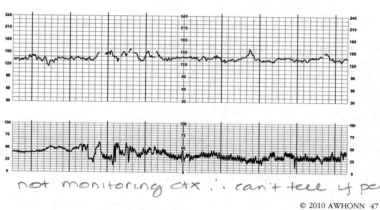

not monitoring ctx ∴ can't tell if periodic changes

© 2010 AWHONN 47

Baseline 130,
Variability moderate = 6-25 bpm
CAT I tracing normal at this time

Systematic Assessment
of FHR Tracings

STEP 1
- Baseline rate

- Variability   primary indicator of fetal oxygenation
  Key to evaluate other components of tracing

- Periodic/episodic changes

- Uterine activity

(Adapted from Fox, Kilpatrick, King, & Parer, 2000)

© 2010 AWHONN 48

Systematic Assessment of FHR Tracings (cont.)

- Pattern evolution

- Accompanying clinical characteristics

- Normalcy vs. urgency

(Adapted from Fox, Kilpatrick, King, & Parer, 2000)

© 2010 AWHONN 49

TO ASSESS

Baseline FHR

The approximate mean FHR rounded to increments of <u>5 bpm</u> during a <u>10-minute</u> window, excluding:

- Accelerations and decelerations
- Periods of marked variability (>25 bpm)

✓ *TEST Q.*

There must be <u>at least 2 minutes</u> of identifiable baseline segments (<u>not necessarily contiguous</u>) in a 10-minute window, or the baseline for that period is <u>indeterminate</u>.

© 2010 AWHONN 50

Baseline FHR (cont.)

- *Normal range:* 110–160 bpm

  (not a decel)
- *Bradycardia:* a baseline of <110 bpm for ≥ 10 minutes

  > 2 & < 10 mins = prolonged decel.

  < 2 = late, variable, early decel
- *Tachycardia:* a baseline of >160 bpm for ≥ 10 minutes

© 2010 AWHONN 51

Baseline FHR Variability

- Fluctuations in the baseline FHR that are irregular in amplitude and frequency
- Quantified as the amplitude of the peak-trough in bpm
- Amplitude range is **visually** quantified as follows:
  - *Absent* FHR variability = undetectable amplitude range = straight/flat l
  - *Minimal* FHR variability = > undetectable ≤ 5 bpm
  - *Moderate* FHR variability = 6–25 bpm amplitude range
  - *Marked* FHR variability = >25 bpm amplitude range

TEST Q ✓

VARIABILITY

© 2010 AWHONN 52

Variability

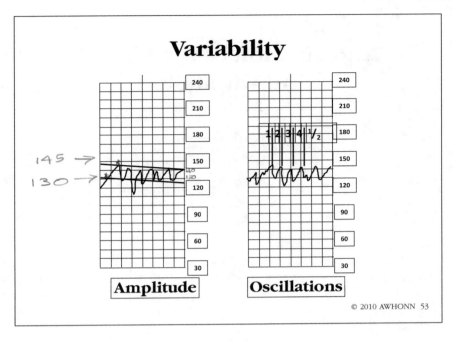

145 →
130 →

Amplitude   **Oscillations**

© 2010 AWHONN 53

Hints for Interpreting Variability

- Three "Ss": THAT AFFECT VARIABILITY

  - Sleep

  - Sedation e.g. epidural, demerol, opiates.
    for pain
    CNS depression.
    • MEDS ↓ MgSO₄ should not ⟹ MINIMUM
      have decels. VARIABILITY
  - Sick should have
    injury to CNS accels
    before admission
    HOL+D
    • SMOKING
    • HYPOGLYCEMIA

© 2010 AWHONN 54

• IMMATURE PARASYMPATHETIC
• CHEMICAL SUBSTANCES/DRUGS.

Regulation of the FHR and Variability

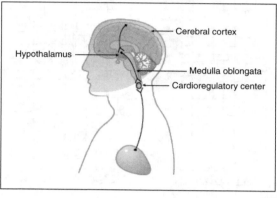

© 2010 AWHONN 55

ABSENT VARIABILITY indicates fetus loses ability to compensate

✓ TEST Q development of fetal acidemia generally occurs c̄ recurrent decels > 1 hr period. c̄ minimal variability

RECURRENT = if occurring c̄ > 50% of ctx

TEST Q ✓

° TO DETERMINE IF TRUE SLEEP CYCLE

- SCALP STIM.

- VIBROACOUSTIC

- BEEPER/VIBRATE.

- ABDOMINAL PALPATION

Moderate Variability

predicts absence of fetal acidemia at the time it's observed

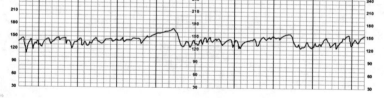

© 2010 AWHONN 56

good oxygenation of fetus, CNS intact

Absent Variability

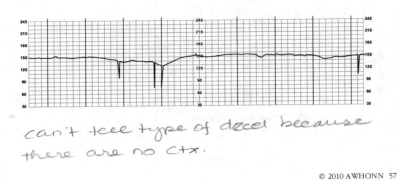

flat line

can't tell type of decel because there are no ctx.

ABSENT VARIABILITY may be caused by TACHYSYSTOLE.

Variability?

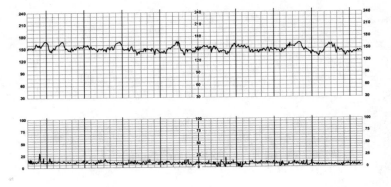

MODERATE VARIABILITY = good oxygenation

Variability? (cont.)

MINIMAL VARIABILITY.

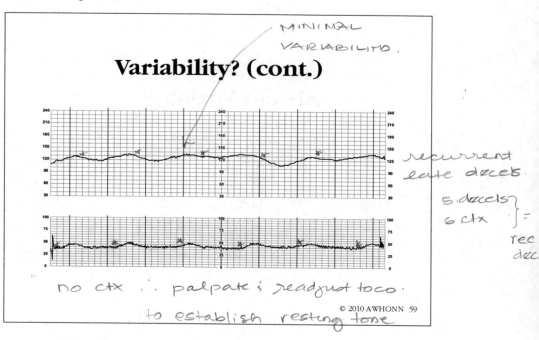

recurrent late decels.

5 decels, 6 ctx } = rec dec

no ctx ∴ palpate & readjust toco. to establish resting tone

© 2010 AWHONN 59

Variability? (cont.)

ABSENT VARIABILITY

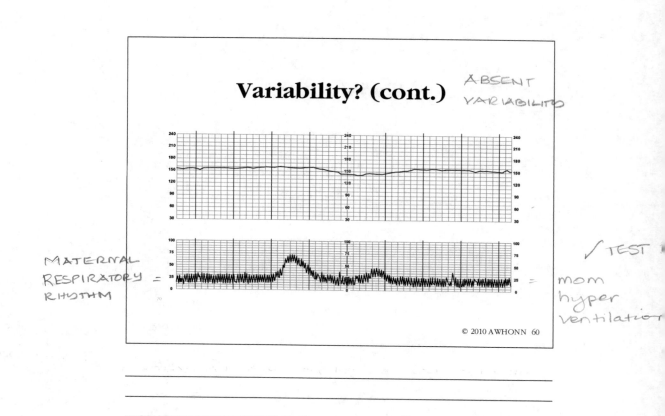

MATERNAL RESPIRATORY RHYTHM =

√ TEST

= mom hyper ventilation

© 2010 AWHONN 60

FHR Auscultation

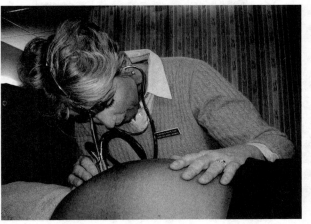

© 2010 AWHONN 61

FETOSCOPE for assessing arrythmia.

in the USA <u>only for</u> *low risk or* <u>normal pts. 1:1 RN to pt ratio</u>, *auscultation of 30 mins i.e. counting the beats.*

<u>if high risk pt then use EFM</u>

Helga (cont.): After Shower

↑ACCEL

TACHO CARDIAC.

FHR 165.

VARIABILITY BASELINE MODERATE

ACCELS.

∅ decels

unable to determine ctx

ctx after readjustment.

palpate then readjustment

© 2010 AWHONN 62

TEST ✓ Q

ASSESS REASON FOR TACHOCARDIA
- take temp
- hot water in shower

<u>if FHR = 165 can no longer use auscultation</u>
<u>must use EFM</u>

reactive strip = 15-30 mins

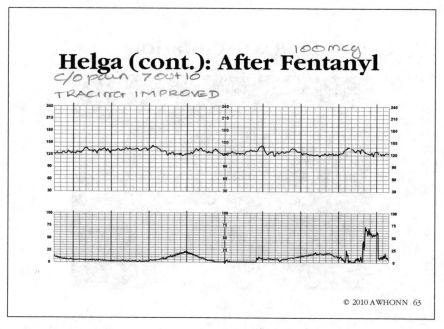

Helga (cont.): After Fentanyl

100 mcg
c/o pain 7 out 10
TRACING IMPROVED

© 2010 AWHONN 63

higher baseline due to maternal pain
from release of catecholamines (intrinsic
factor), not afebrile & pain controlled
can now return to auscultation

Accelerations

- Visually apparent abrupt (onset to peak in < 30 seconds) increases in FHR above the baseline
- In fetus ≥ 32 weeks, peak ≥ 15 bpm and last for ≥ 15 seconds from onset to return to baseline
- In fetus < 32 weeks, peak ≥ 10 bpm and last for ≥ 10 seconds from onset to return to baseline
- *Prolonged* acceleration is ≥ 2 minutes but < 10 minutes in duration
- Indicate **normal fetal acid–base** status

© 2010 AWHONN 64

ACCELS IN
° FULLTERM FETUS
- 15 × 15

° ACCELS IN
PRETERM FETUS
- 10 × 10

10 beats by 10 sec

minimal variability ē accel = baby sleeping

MODERATE { adequate O₂ to brain
VARIABILITY { CNS intact

onset · nadir

→ lowest point of decel

Decelerations

Type	Definition: Visually Apparent Decrease in FHR
Early	***Gradual*** onset: ≥ 30 sec from onset to nadir; nadir simultaneous with peak of contraction
Late	***Gradual*** onset: ≥ 30 sec from onset to nadir; delayed in timing—nadir after peak of contraction
Variable	***Abrupt*** onset: < 30 sec from onset to beginning of nadir, lasting ≥ 15 sec but < 2 min; depth ≥ 15 bpm
Prolonged	Decrease of ≥ 15 bpm lasting ≥ 2 min but less than 10 min (≥ 10 min = baseline change)

© 2010 AWHONN 65

= MIRROR IMAGE OF Ctx due to head compression ∴ CNS intact
= starts & ends after ctx

= VARIABLES: can occur before, during or after ctx

✓ TEST Q

VARIABLES - MUST BE ABRUPT,

MEMORIZE ✓ TEST Q.

Periodic vs. Episodic
Recurrent vs. Intermittent

- *Periodic:* associated with uterine contractions.
- *Episodic:* not associated with uterine contractions.   e.g. variable, but not late decels
- *Recurrent:* decelerations that occur with ≥ 50% of uterine contractions within a 20-minute period.
- *Intermittent:* decelerations that occur with < 50% of uterine contractions within a 20-minute period.

© 2010 AWHONN 66

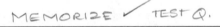

Uterine Activity

- *Normal:* ≤ 5 contractions in 10 minutes, averaged over a 30-minute window

- *Tachysystole:* > 5 contractions in 10 minutes, averaged over a 30-minute window

uterus not getting an opportunity to relax
↳INTERVENTIONS
terbutaline
hydration

Macones et al., 2008

© 2010 AWHONN 67

Interpretation of FHR Patterns

- Three Tier FHR Interpretation System:
  - Category I—predicts normal acid–base status
  - Category II—indeterminate
  - Category III—predicts abnormal acid–base status

Macones et al., 2008

© 2010 AWHONN 68

RECURRENT DECELS >1 late decel due to uteroplacental insufficiency
due to
- overstimulation
- htn

Category I—Normal FHR Tracing

- Includes <u>ALL</u> of the following:
  - Baseline FHR: 110–160 bpm
  - Baseline variability: moderate
  - Late or variable decelerations: absent *i.e. more than one variable decel*
  - Early decelerations: present or absent
  - Accelerations: present or absent
- Predictive of normal fetal acid–base status *@ the time of interpretation*
- Followed in routine manner *i.e. allow maternal fetal oxygenation*

↓ pain
↑ position

Macones et al., 2008

© 2010 AWHONN 69

Category II—Indeterminate FHR Tracing

- Includes <u>**ALL tracings**</u> not categorized as Category I or Category III
- Category II tracings are indeterminate:
  - <u>Not</u> predictive of abnormal fetal acid–base status
  - Not enough evidence to classify as I or III
- Warrant evaluation, surveillance and reevaluation:
  - This does not mean "no action"

Macones et al., 2008

© 2010 AWHONN 70

RECURRENT DECELS >1

Category II—Indeterminate (cont.)

- Will include many tracings encountered in clinical care
- Some <u>examples</u>:
  - Bradycardia not accompanied by absent variability
  - Tachycardia
  - Minimal baseline variability
  - Absence of induced accelerations after fetal stimulation
  - Prolonged decelerations
  - Recurrent late decelerations with moderate variability

Macones et al., 2008

© 2010 AWHONN 71

Category II—Indeterminate (cont.)

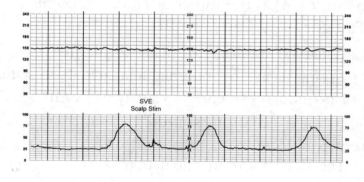

© 2010 AWHONN 72

Category II—Indeterminate (cont.)

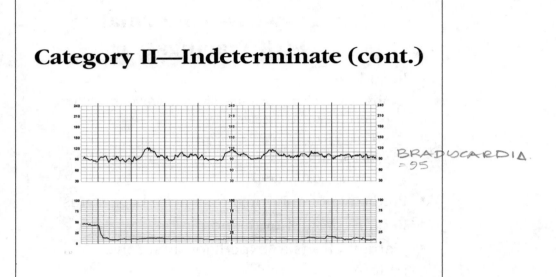

BRADYCARDIA
= 95

Category II—Indeterminate (cont.)

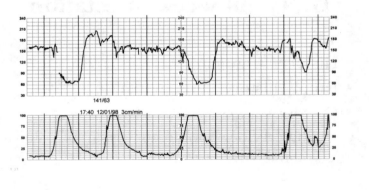

141/63

17:40 12/01/98 3cm/min

could be due to
- cord compression
- oligo
- fully dilated

warrants exam

Category III—Abnormal FHR Tracings

- Include *either:*
  - Absent baseline FHR variability and any of the following:
    - Recurrent late decelerations
    - Recurrent variable decelerations
    - Bradycardia
  - or a sinusoidal pattern
- Predictive of abnormal fetal acid–base status
- Require prompt evaluation
- Warrant efforts to expeditiously resolve pattern

© 2010 AWHONN 75

Latoya, 17 Years Old
G_1, P_0, 38 Weeks' Gestation

- History: unremarkable
- Family history: unremarkable
- Current status:
  - SROM 1 hour prior to admission, occasional contractions

T = 98.5°

© 2010 AWHONN 76

Latoya (cont.)

Current pregnancy:

- Prenatal course uncomplicated
- 12 prenatal visits
- Two ultrasounds confirmed date and size

© 2010 AWHONN 77

RISK FACTORS   17y/o, ROM, nutritional status,

TO ASSESS TRACING

1. Baseline
2. Variability
3. periodic or
   episodic
   patterns

Latoya (cont.): Admission Tracing

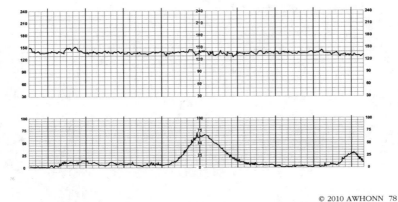

© 2010 AWHONN 78

PLAN.
- continue to
  monitor
  i.e expectant
  mgmt.

Baseline = 135   VARIABILITY = moderate CAT 1
Accels   = 15 X 15

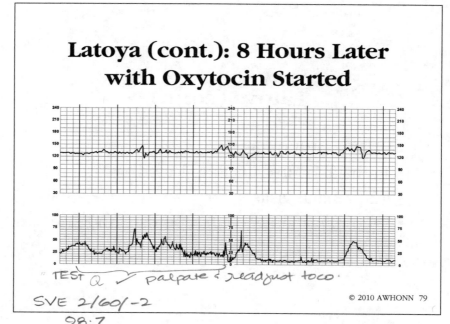

Latoya (cont.): 8 Hours Later with Oxytocin Started

© 2010 AWHONN 79

TEST @ ✓ *palpate & readjust toco.*

SVE 2/60/-2

98·7

BASELINE = 135   ACCEL , Ø decel because not 15×15

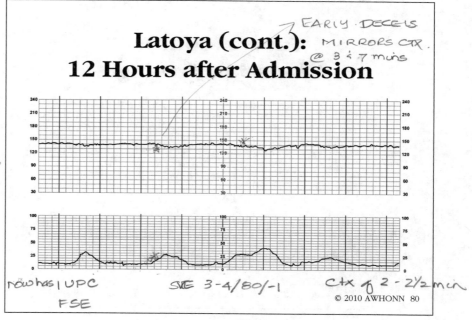

Latoya (cont.): 12 Hours after Admission

EARLY DECELS
MIRRORS CTX.
@ 3 & 7 mins

FSE used if
– can't assess
fetal heart rate
– obese pt

now has 1 UPC
FSE

SVE 3–4/80/-1   Ctx of 2 – 2½ min

© 2010 AWHONN 80

IUPC – for
intensity
of ctx.

Baseline 140 , MINIMAL VARIABILITY

VARIABILITY due to sympathetic & parasympathetic systems.

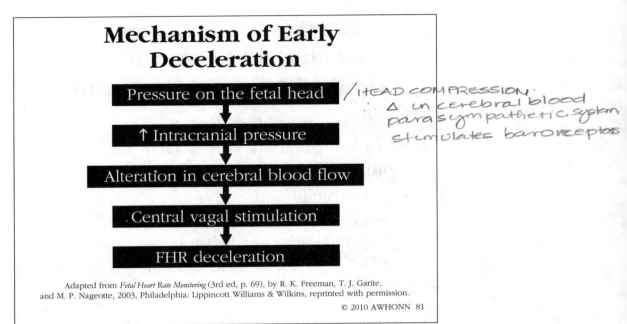

Mechanism of Early Deceleration

Pressure on the fetal head

↓

↑ Intracranial pressure

↓

Alteration in cerebral blood flow

↓

Central vagal stimulation

↓

FHR deceleration

Adapted from *Fetal Heart Rate Monitoring* (3rd ed, p. 69), by R. K. Freeman, T. J. Garite, and M. P. Nageotte, 2003, Philadelphia: Lippincott Williams & Wilkins, reprinted with permission.

© 2010 AWHONN 81

↑ HEAD COMPRESSION:
∴ Δ in cerebral blood
parasympathetic system
stimulates baroreceptors

LOOK AT EVOLUTION OF TRACING
to determine how it changed

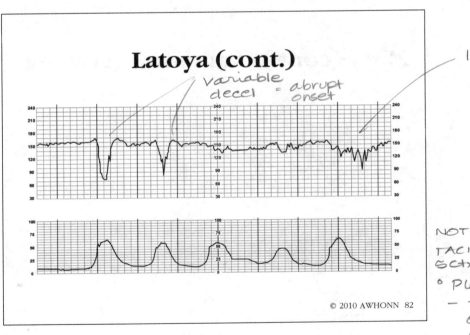

Latoya (cont.)

variable decel = abrupt onset

late decel.

© 2010 AWHONN 82

NOT
TACHYSYSTOLE.
5 ctx in 9 min period
° PLAN
— turn pitocin
off because of
baseline change
& 5 ctx in 9 min
period.

Baseline 160, variable & late decels.

C section in 30 min
APGAR expected 7, 9

Mary, 30 Years Old
G_1, P_0, 38 Weeks' Gestation

- History: unremarkable
- Current pregnancy: prenatal period unremarkable
- In hospital:
  - Spontaneous rupture of membranes 2 hours prior to admission
  - 98°F (36.7°C) temperature, other vital signs within normal limits

© 2010 AWHONN 83

RISK FACTORS - infection due to SROM

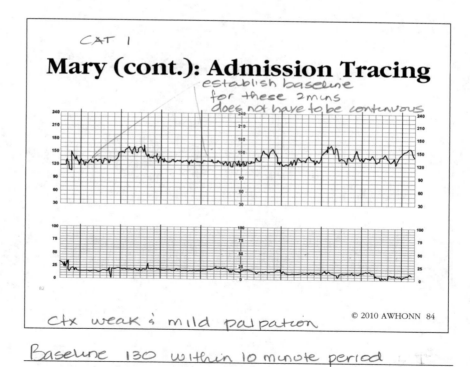

CAT 1

Mary (cont.): Admission Tracing

establish baseline for these 2 mins does not have to be continuous

© 2010 AWHONN 84

PLAN intermittent mgmt

Ctx weak & mild palpation

Baseline 130 within 10 minute period

Mary (cont.): EFM Reapplied

* abrupt onset

variable =

< 30 sec from start to end

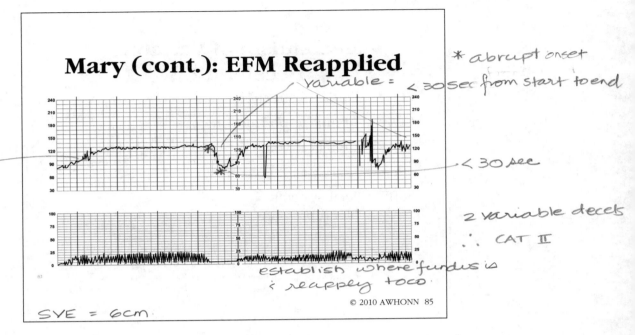

< 30 sec

2 variable decels
∴ CAT II

establish where fundus is
& reapply toco.

© 2010 AWHONN 85

SVE = 6cm.

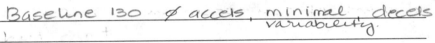

Baseline 130 Ø accels, minimal decels
variability.

Mary (cont.): Toco Readjusted

Variable decels. = abrupt onset

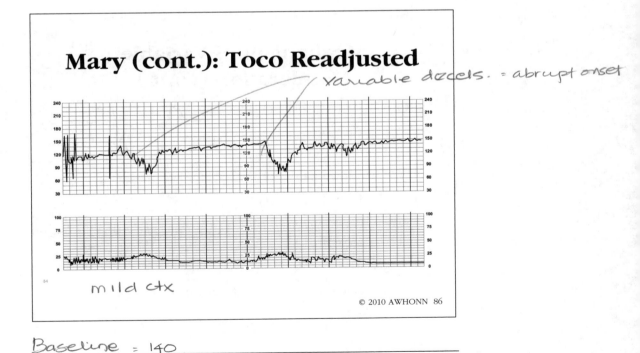

mild ctx

© 2010 AWHONN 86

Baseline = 140

○ UMBILICAL CORD.

- 2 ARTERIES

- 1 VEIN
  (lumen softer
  than artery)

Mechanism of Variable Deceleration

PO = Partial obstruction

CO = Complete obstruction

UV = Umbilical vein occluded fast
=> ↓ fetal BP = hypotension => sympathetic nervous system.

UA = Umbilical artery ↑ FHR

FSBP = Fetal systemic blood pressure

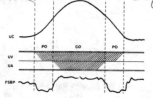

(Reprinted with permission from the American College of Obstetricians and Gynecologists [*Obstetrics and Gynecology*, 1975, *45*(2), p. 145, Wolters Kluwer Health]).

© 2010 AWHONN 87

at peak of ctx occlusion of all vessels.
no O₂ coming in, no CO₂ going out. Triggers
baroreceptors => stimulate parasympathetic
↓ FHR
once compression releases recovery occurs.
if fetus comprised, doesn't rebound

Mechanism of Variable Deceleration (cont.)

PO = Partial obstruction

CO = Complete obstruction

UV = Umbilical vein

UA = Umbilical artery

FSBP = Fetal systemic blood pressure

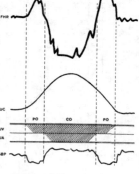

(Reprinted with permission from the American College of Obstetricians and Gynecologists [*Obstetrics and Gynecology*, 1975, *45*(2), p. 145, Wolters Kluwer Health])

© 2010 AWHONN 88

RECURRENT VARIABLES:
occur ≧ 50% of ctx
over 30 min period

Student Materials | **65**

Mary (cont.):
Tracing of Variable Shapes

= most frequently seen.

RELIEVE CORD COMPRESSION
Δ position

↳ OLIGOHYDRAMNIOS OR SROM
⇒ keep cord floating
amnioinfusion

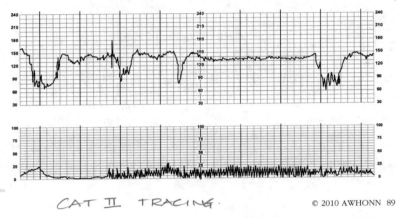

CAT II TRACING.

© 2010 AWHONN 89

Baseline 135

○ ANALYZE PH (oxygenation)
1. fetal pulse ox

2. fetal scalp sampling

Fetal Pulse Oximetry Tracing

to analyze fetal oxygenation.

FSpO2 44%   FSpO2 41%   FSpO2 44%   FSpO2 44%

© 2010 AWHONN 90

30% threshold i.e. metabolic acidosis
does not develop until saturation falls
below 30% for 10-15 min

Normal fetal oxygenation in labor = 30-65%

2nd stage of labor

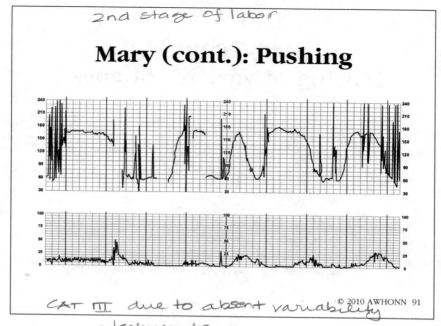

Mary (cont.): Pushing

© 2010 AWHONN 91

CAT III due to absent variability

= tachycardic

Baseline 170   Minimal → absent, recurrent deep variables

expeditious delivery. Fetus reserve is

stressed i not recovering adequately.

NSVD   expected apgars 3, 5, 7

3 = fetus had metabolic acidosis.

UTERO PLACENTAL INSUFFICIENCY.

can't adequately supply baby's needs.

Mary (cont.): Outcome

- Baby girl

- Outlet forceps delivery

- Apgar scores 3/5/7

- True knot in the cord

© 2010 AWHONN 92

Rita, 26 Years Old
G_1, P_0, 40 2/7 Weeks' Gestation

Family history:

- Maternal grandmother: hypertension

- Maternal grandfather: cardiac disease

- Father of baby in good health

© 2010 AWHONN 93

RISK FACTORS - family hx of htn, ♡ disease
fetus may have cardiac disease, watch BPs.
past due date @ 40^{+2}
↓ AFV in past due dates

Rita (cont.)

- Medical history:
  - Exercise-induced asthma
  - Irritable bowel syndrome
- Current pregnancy:
  - Routine prenatal care
  - Prenatal labs: normal values

© 2010 AWHONN 94

RISK FACTORS   exercise induced asthma.

Rita (cont.): Admission Tracing

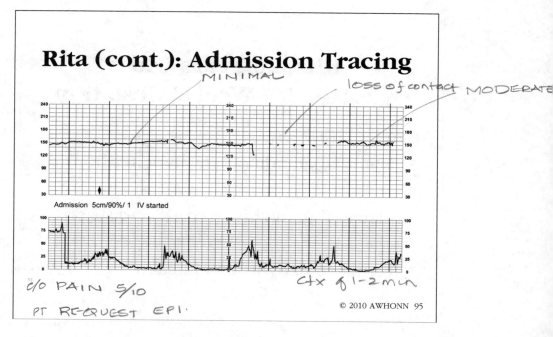

MINIMAL

loss of contact MODERATE

Admission 5cm/90%/ 1 IV started

c/o PAIN 5/10

PT REQUEST EPI.

Ctx q 1-2min

© 2010 AWHONN 95

Baseline 155   MINIMAL - MODERATE VARIABILITY.

Rita (cont.): Post-epidural

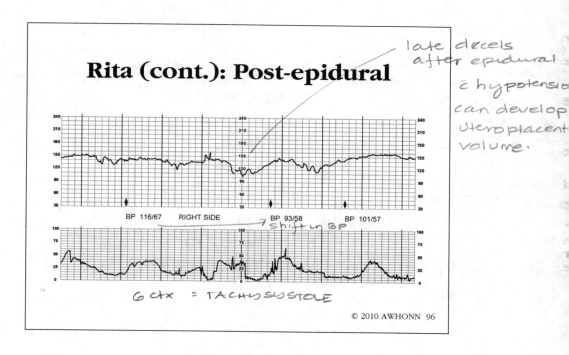

late decels
after epidural.
c̄ hypotensio
can develop
Uteroplacent
volume.

BP 116/67   RIGHT SIDE   BP 93/58   BP 101/57

shift in BP

6 ctx = TACHYSYSTOLE

© 2010 AWHONN 96

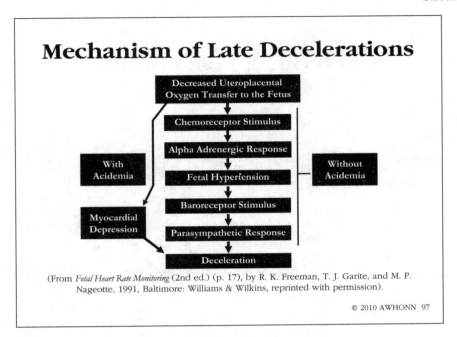

Mechanism of Late Decelerations

Decreased Uteroplacental Oxygen Transfer to the Fetus

Chemoreceptor Stimulus

Alpha Adrenergic Response

Fetal Hypertension

Baroreceptor Stimulus

Parasympathetic Response

Deceleration

With Acidemia

Without Acidemia

Myocardial Depression

(From *Fetal Heart Rate Monitoring* (2nd ed.) (p. 17), by R. K. Freeman, T. J. Garite, and M. P. Nageotte, 1991, Baltimore: Williams & Wilkins, reprinted with permission).

© 2010 AWHONN 97

fetal respond to ↓ O₂ by releasing catecholamines
⇒ peripheral vasoconstriction shunts
blood to brain, heart, adrenals.
2 recurrent decles may develop NEC.
because blood is shunted away from gut

RECURRENT LATE č MINIMAL ⇒ fetal acidemia
                    VARIABILITY

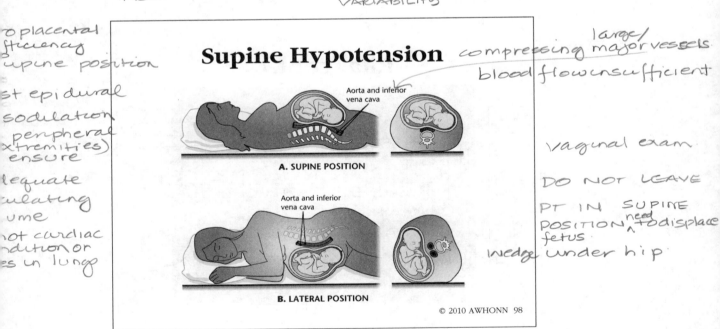

o placental
fficiency
upine position

st epidural
sodilation
   peripheral
xtremities)
ensure

lequate
ulating
ume

ot cardiac
dition or
es in lungs

Supine Hypotension

compressing large/major vessels
blood flow insufficient

Aorta and inferior vena cava

A. SUPINE POSITION

Aorta and inferior vena cava

B. LATERAL POSITION

vaginal exam.

DO NOT LEAVE
PT IN SUPINE
POSITION, need to displace
fetus.
wedge under hip

© 2010 AWHONN 98

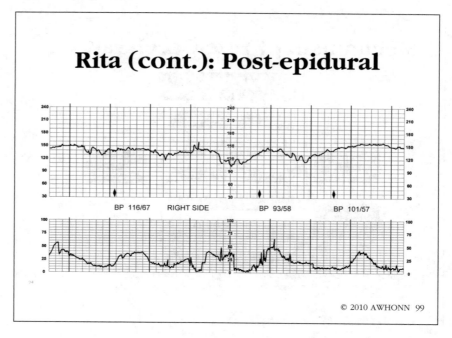

changed position

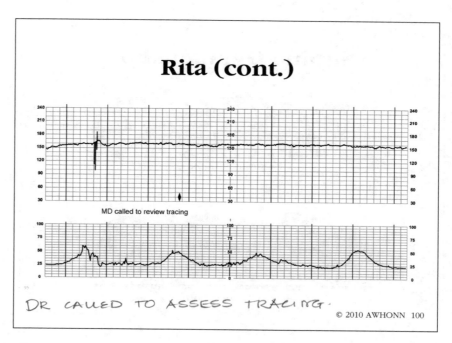

Baseline 160 MINIMAL VARIABILITY
FORCEPS DELIVERY
EXPECTED APGAR 2, 6, 7

Jane, 40 Years Old
G_3, P_{2002}, 42 Weeks' Gestation

- History:
  - Poor nutritional status
  - Two living children, delivered vaginally at 40 and 41 weeks, respectively
- Current pregnancy:
  - Three prenatal visits
  - Smokes ½ pack of cigarettes per day
  - Poor nutritional status
  - 8 lb (3.6 kg) weight gain

© 2010 AWHONN 101

RISK   AMA, WT GAIN, SMOKING,
        3 PRENATL VISITS,

Jane (cont.)

Current pregnancy:

- Vaginal exam: 2 cm/80%/-1
- Premature rupture of membranes > 12 hours, clear fluid, no odor
- 98.4°F (36.9°C) temperature

© 2010 AWHONN 102

PROM
after 1 hr of ROM
i̇ no ctx

AT RISK FOR INFECTION

Assessing Uterine Activity

- Frequency _or peak to peak of ctx beginning to beginning of ct_
- Duration _how long in sec_
- Intensity _how soft or firm between ctx to determine resting tone_
- Resting tone
- Adequacy of uterine activity _ctx q 2-3 min but not >5 in a min period_

© 2010 AWHONN 103

intensity of contraction measured IUPC mild / moderate strong = can't indent c̄ pressure.

MUST HAVE CTX THAT ARE ADEQUATE

Cervix dilates ; fetus descends

Jane (cont.): Admission Tracing

accels.

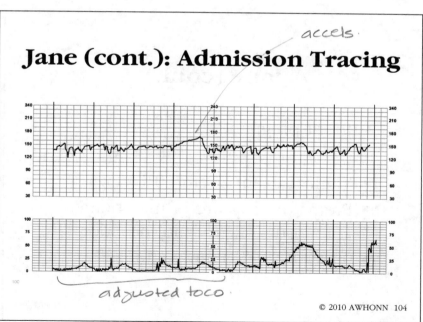

adjusted toco.

© 2010 AWHONN 104

TO MONITOR FOR CHORIO

99.0°F monitor temp every hr.

BASELINE = MODERATE VARIABILITY C̄ ACCELS
RISK FOR CHORIO C̄ ROM > 12 HRS.

Jane (cont.):
12 Hours after Admission

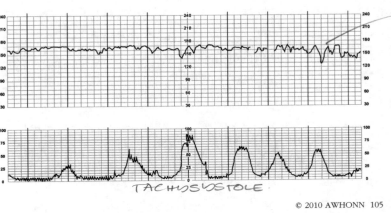

decels

TACHYSYSTOLE

© 2010 AWHONN 105

21 HRS AT ROM > 12 HRS
BASELINE 165   MODERATE VARIABILITY

Jane (cont.):
(1½ Hours Later—13½ Hours
after Admission)

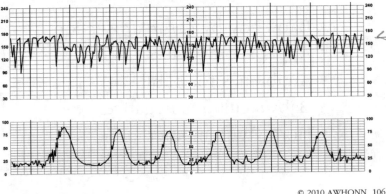

MARKED
VARIABILITY.
fetus attempting
to compensate.
when can no
longer compensate

© 2010 AWHONN 106

PLAN.
1. PITOCIN OFF

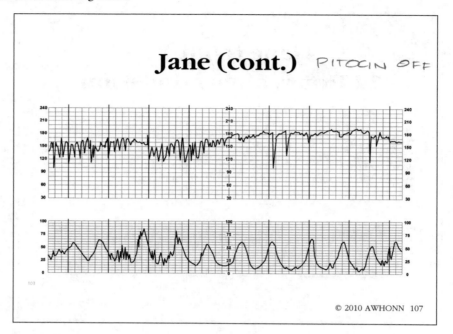

Jane (cont.) PITOCIN OFF

© 2010 AWHONN 107

BASELINE ↑ TO 180, TEMP ↑

PLAN TERB BECAUSE AT 4CM (REMOTE FROM DELIVERY)

PITOCIN
- has short ½ life
- take 10-12 mins for ½ of pit to be degraded

Jane (cont.): Outcome

- Baby boy by <u>cesarean section</u>
- Apgar scores 5/7/8
- Antibiotics for baby
- Baby's cultures negative
- Home with mother

© 2010 AWHONN 108

Oxytocin Administration Based on the Cumulative Body of Physiologic and Pharmacologic Evidence

© 2010 AWHONN 109

Oxytocin as High-Alert Medication

- Institute for Safe Medication Practices designated IV oxytocin as a high-alert medication in 2007.

- Medication errors involving IV oxytocin are dose-related and commonly involve excessive uterine activity with subsequent fetal response.

© 2010 AWHONN 110

Oxytocin as High-Alert Medication (cont.)

Standard care processes for oxytocin administration are recommended to enhance safety when this medication is used.

© 2010 AWHONN 111

Endogenous Oxytocin

from POSTERIOR PITUIT
in a pulsatile manner

- First stage of labor:
  - Maternal circulating concentrations approximately = 2 to 4 mU/min
- Fetal contribution:
  - Secretion similar to 3 mU/min
- Combined effects = 5 to 7 mU/min
- Second stage of labor: *when fetus is descending*
  - Surge of oxytocin at Ferguson's reflex

© 2010 AWHONN 112

Response to Exogenous Oxytocin

- Initial incremental phase (1.5 to 2 hours):
  - Uterine contractions will progressively increase in frequency and intensity.
- Stable phase (3.5 to 4.5 hours):
  - Any further increase will not cause more frequent normal changes in uterine activity but may result in side effects (tachysystole/unfavorable FHR response).

© 2010 AWHONN 113

Response to Exogenous Oxytocin (cont.)

- Oxytocin receptor sites decrease significantly during prolonged oxytocin-induced or augmented labor compared to spontaneous labor.
- Desensitization is related to dosage rate and length of administration.
- More oxytocin for dysfunctional labor will cause further desensitization.
- A rest period of 1–2 hours is recommended.

(Phaneuf et al., 2000)

© 2010 AWHONN 114

Pharmacokinetics

- Half-life 10 to 12 minutes
- Three to four half-lives are needed to reach steady-state plasma concentration
- Full effect of oxytocin cannot be evaluated until steady-state concentration has been achieved
- Basis for recommendations for 30- to 40-minute interval dosing of oxytocin

IDEALLY turn putocin up q 30-40 minutes

© 2010 AWHONN 115

Oxytocin Dosage

- Based on the evidence:
  - Physiologic dose is best:
    - 90% of women will achieve active labor at less than 6 mU/min.
    - Most women do not need more than 10 mU/min.
    - Lowest possible dose to achieve physiologic effect.
  - At least 30–40 minutes between increases is optimal.
  - No data exists that more oxytocin will improve dysfunctional labor.

Crane & Young (1998); Daniel-Spiegel et al. (2004); Phaneuf et al. (2000); Simpson (2008)

© 2010 AWHONN 116

° TACHYSYSTOLE

- stop pit
- alert MD

- terb ready

- OR set up

establish 200 - 220 MVU.
ctx q 2-3 mins, lasting 80-90 sec, allowing
the uterus to rest ; palpate ctx — mild, moderate, strong

Oxytocin Dosage (cont.)

Based on the evidence:

- Continuing oxytocin after active labor is established will not shorten labor.
- Long duration and high dose may have opposite the intended effects on the course of labor by desensitizing uterine receptors to exogenous and endogenous oxytocin.
- Labor is generally self-sustaining once the active phase is established.

Evidence-Based Protocol

- Start at 1 mU/min
- Increase by 1–2 mU/min every 30 to 40 min
- Contractions every 2–3 min
- Labor progress
- Active labor: decrease dose or discontinue
- Titrate to fetal and uterine response
- Avoid tachysystole; treat before undesired FHR response develops

Strategies for Minimizing Risk of Harm

- Standardized process for oxytocin administration:
  - Elective labor induction only after 39 weeks of gestation
  - Standard protocols and/or order sets based on current physiologic and pharmacologic evidence
  - Standard concentration of oxytocin prepared by pharmacy

(Simpson, 2008; Simpson & Knox, 2009)

© 2010 AWHONN 119

Strategies for Minimizing Risk of Harm (cont.)

- Standard definition of desired effect of oxytocin administration
- Standard definition of uterine tachysystole
- Standard treatment of oxytocin-induced uterine tachysystole guided by fetal status

© 2010 AWHONN 120

Strategies for Minimizing Risk of Harm (cont.)

- Methods to mitigate harm that may result from error:
  - Protocols that allow discontinuing or decreasing the dose without contacting the physician or nurse midwife
  - Consensus rescue protocols available

(Simpson, 2008; Simpson & Knox, 2009)

© 2010 AWHONN 121

Tina, 26 Years Old
G_1, P_0, 39 Weeks' Gestation

- History: unremarkable

© 2010 AWHONN 122

Tina (cont.)

Current pregnancy:
- 15 prenatal visits
- 30 lb (13.6 kg) weight gain
- SROM at 0650, clear fluid, no odor
- Vaginal exam: 5 cm/100%/0
- Vital signs WNL: T 98°F (36.7°C)

© 2010 AWHONN 123

RISK FACTORS   SROM

CAT II

Tina (cont.): Admission Tracing at 0719

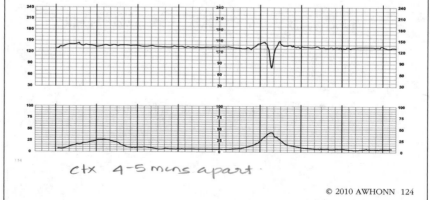

ctx 4-5 mins apart.

© 2010 AWHONN 124

o PLAN
— LEOPOLD'S MANUEVER
— scalp stim
⇒ accel

determine when pattern started
possible sleep cycle
MINIMAL VARIABILITY

rebreather mask
100% O_2

cannula
% O_2

ple mask
- 40%

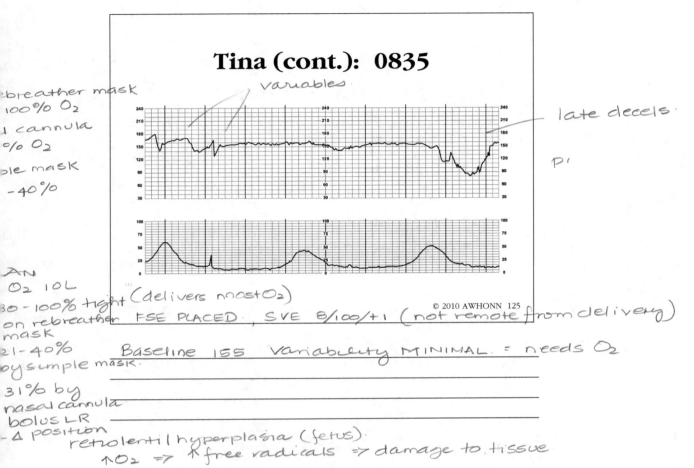

Tina (cont.): 0835

variables

late decels.

Pi

AN
O_2 10L
30 - 100% tight (delivers most O_2)
on rebreather   FSE PLACED, SVE 8/100/+1 (not remote from delivery)
mask
21 - 40%
by simple mask.   Baseline 155 Variability MINIMAL. = needs O_2

31% by
nasal cannula
bolus LR
- Δ position   retrolentil hyperplasia (fetus).
        ↑O_2 ⇒ ↑free radicals ⇒ damage to tissue

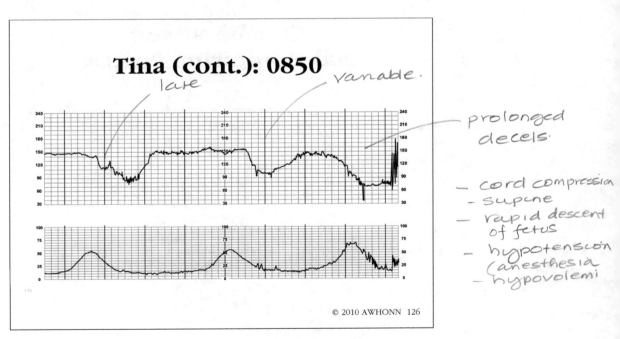

Tina (cont.): 0850

late

variable.

prolonged
decels.

- cord compression
- supine
- rapid descent
  of fetus
- hypotension
  (anesthesia
- hypovolemi

MODERATE VARIABILITY

Tina (cont.): Outcome

- Baby boy by cesarean section
- Apgar scores 8/9
- Tight nuchal cord ×1
- 20% abruption
- Cord gases within normal limits

© 2010 AWHONN 127

Collaborative
Fetal Monitoring Process

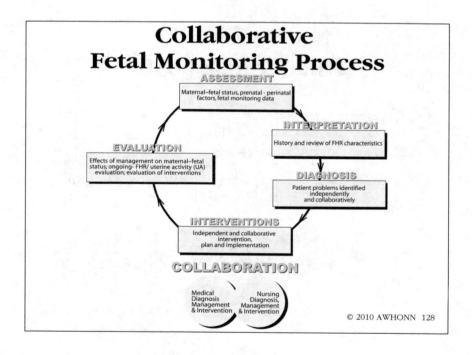

© 2010 AWHONN 128

Techniques of Fetal Heart Monitoring

FHR and UA Monitoring

- Most women in the United States and Canada undergo continuous EFM during labor.

- Knowledge about ALL methods of FHR and UA monitoring is necessary.

Benefits and Limitations of Techniques

Method	Benefits	Limitations
Auscultation	Noninvasive; high touch; widespread application	1:1 staffing; technical difficulty; FHR variability not assessed
Palpation	Noninvasive; high touch; widespread application	Subjectivity; intrauterine pressure subjectively assessed
Ultrasound	Noninvasive; continuous FHR signal achievable	Signal strength varies; may restrict movement; EFM associated with ↑intervention rates
Tocodynamometer	Noninvasive; continuous UA recording achievable	Does not detect intrauterine pressure; signal strength varies
Fetal spiral electrode	Continuous FHR signal achievable	Invasive; potential risk of infection; may record MHR in fetal demise
Intrauterine pressure catheter	Continuous UA signal; intrauterine resting tone, contraction pressure measured	Invasive; ↑ risk for infection, uterine perforation, abruption; readings sensitive to position changes

© 2010 AWHONN 131

Margaret, 23 Years Old
G_1, P_0, 401/7 Weeks' Gestation

- History: unremarkable

- Current pregnancy:
  - + Group B Strep by urine culture at 36 weeks' gestation
  - 61 lb (27.7 kg) pregnancy weight gain

watch BP.

© 2010 AWHONN 132

Margaret (cont.): Labor Admission

- Admission for oxytocin induction @ 6AM
- Vital signs: BP 110/62, P 94, T 97.5°F (36.4°C)
- Vaginal exam: 4 cm/90%/-1 station
- Membranes intact
- Method of monitoring:
  - Auscultation and palpation until resources stabilize

© 2010 AWHONN 133

Intermittent Auscultation

- Intermittent counting of the FHR with a fetoscope or handheld Doppler ultrasound:
  - Fetoscope detects heart sounds.
  - Doppler detects reflected sound from heart motion.
- Fetoscope can be used for troubleshooting:
  - Verification of FHR arrhythmias
  - Clarification of maternal vs fetal FHR, or halving or doubling of the FHR on the EFM tracing
- Allows women freedom of movement

© 2010 AWHONN 134

Benefits of Auscultation

- Recommended nurse-to-patient staff ratio is 1:1
- Increased hands-on time with patient:
  - Cannot be accomplished indirectly
- Neonatal outcomes compare favorably with EFM

© 2010 AWHONN 135

Limitations of Auscultation

- FHR assessment may be limited by position or movement of mother and fetus, maternal size or uterine tension.
- 1:1 nurse–patient ratio may require staffing realignment.
- Auscultation requires education, practice and skill.
- Auscultation is not continuous.
- Fetal heart rate variability and types of decelerations may not be assessed.
- No copy generated for collaborative decision making and record keeping.

© 2010 AWHONN 136

Interpreting Auscultation Findings

Category I—Normal Auscultation Findings— Predictive of Fetal Well-being
Includes **ALL** of the following: • Normal FHR baseline between 110–160 bpm • Regular rhythm • Presence of FHR increases or accelerations from the baseline • Absence of FHR decreases or decelerations from the baseline
Category II—Indeterminate Auscultation Findings
Includes **ANY** of the following: • Irregular rhythm • Presence of FHR decreases or decelerations from the baseline • Tachycardia (baseline > 160 bpm> 10 minutes in duration) • Bradycardia (baseline < 110 bpm> 10 minutes in duration)

© 2010 AWHONN 137

_____

_____

_____

_____

Margaret (cont.)

Auscultation Findings
- Rate: 130s–140s (RANGE)
- Rhythm: regular
- Increases in FHR to 150s–170s
- No decreases auscultated

Palpation Findings
- No palpable contractions
- Resting tone soft

© 2010 AWHONN 138

_____

_____

_____

_____

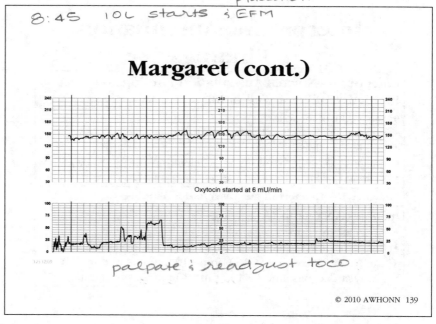

8:45   IOL starts č EFM placed on

Margaret (cont.)

Oxytocin started at 6 mU/min

palpate č readjust toco

© 2010 AWHONN 139

MODERATE VARIABILITY, ACCELS

Doppler Ultrasound Transducer

- Device detects fetal heart movement
- Second-generation monitors and autocorrelation
- Maternal or fetal heart rate?
- Artifact

© 2010 AWHONN 140

Machine Half
and Double Counting

- Greater than 240 bpm

- Less than 30 bpm

- Maternal or fetal heart rate may be halved or double counted under certain conditions

  ∴ check maternal pulse

© 2010 AWHONN 141

Example of Half Counting

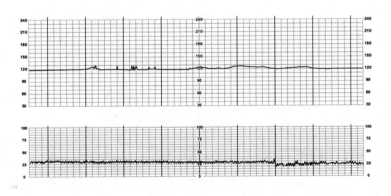

© 2010 AWHONN 142

audio beats out @ 240, assess MHR.
use doppler whenever

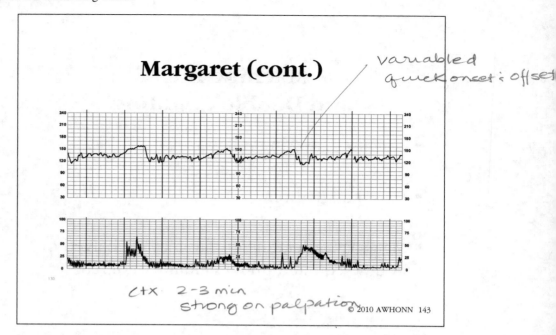

Margaret (cont.)

variable&
quick onset & offset

ctx 2-3 min
strong on palpation

Baseline 135 Variability moderate, accels

2:40 uncomfortable, FSE placed, IUPC placed
because cervix unchanged

Margaret (cont.)

oxytocin ↑

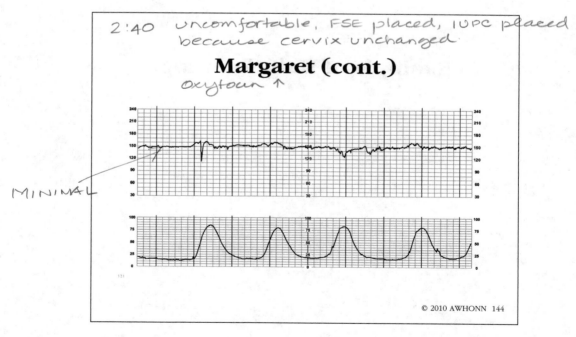

MINIMAL

Baseline 150 changed from 135-150
Do not ↑ pit but ↓ or stop

Fetal Spiral Electrode

- Directly monitors fetal ECG
- Indicated when continuous detection of FHR is clinically necessary and not achievable by US transducer
- Direct conduit for infection—pierces skin on fetal presenting part

© 2010 AWHONN 145

Artifact = irregular variability.

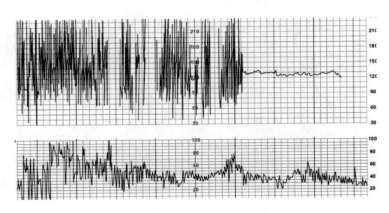

© 2010 AWHONN 146

t arrythmia —use fetoscope,

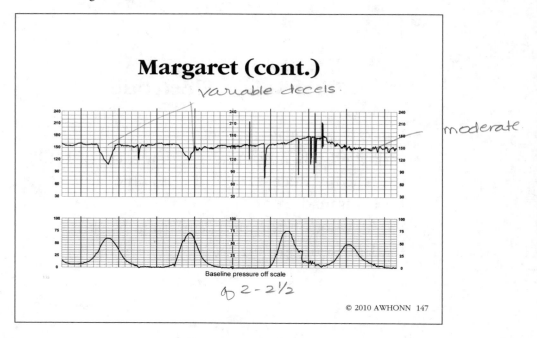

Margaret (cont.)

variable decels

moderate

Baseline pressure off scale

⊕ 2 - 2½

Baseline 150, minimal - moderate variability
continue to monitor, verify ctx pattern

Margaret (cont.): Outcome

- Cesarean birth *due to failure to progress.*
- Male infant
- Birth weight: 9 lb, 11 oz (4,394 g)
- Apgar scores of 8/9 *due to moderate variability*

Pat, 32, Years Old
G$_6$, P$_{3204}$, Weeks' Gestation
Unclear

- History:
  - Chronic hypertension
  - Previous twins died in infancy
- Current pregnancy:
  - No prenatal care *∴ GA of fetus unclear 31-35 wks.*
  - Suspected intrauterine growth restriction (IUGR)
  - Vital signs: BP 134/92, P 80, T 97.5°F (36.4°C)
  - Albumin negative *watch BP.*

© 2010 AWHONN 149

Pat (cont.): Admission Tracing

not an accel

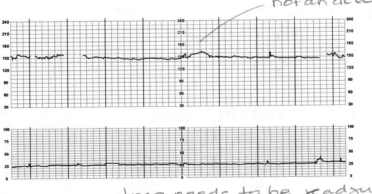

toco needs to be readjusted after palpation

© 2010 AWHONN 150

Baseline 150   Minimal variability

Palpation

- Traditional method of uterine activity assessment in many parts of the world:
  - Frequency, duration, intensity, resting tone
- Importance in assessment and validation of uterine activity should not be underestimated:
  - Palpation of intensity and resting tone an essential component of assessment regardless of monitoring method
- Skills should be verified

© 2010 AWHONN 151

Pat (cont.)

Plan of care:

- Continuous fetal monitoring

- Daily fetal movement count

- Biophysical profile

BPP measures respiratory effect movement

either 2 or 0

© 2010 AWHONN 152

Admitted.

CAT II

Pat (cont.)

prolonged decel < 2 [min] not
> 2 < 10

0 ctx.

© 2010 AWHONN 153

minimal variability

Pat (cont.)

Plan of care:

to determine L:S ratio

- Amniocentesis results: immature lungs

- Steroid dosing

- Continuous electronic fetal monitoring

© 2010 AWHONN 154

Pat (cont.): Day 5

- Amniocentesis mature
- Diastolic BP range: 100–105 mmHg   *intervention*
- Vaginal exam: 2–3 cm/50%/-1
- Continued prolonged decelerations
- Plan: oxytocin induction

© 2010 AWHONN 155

Tocodynamometry

- Pressure-sensitive button translates degree of pressure detected into electrical signal

- Tracing produces relative numbers, not exact information

- Must be used in conjunction with palpation

© 2010 AWHONN 156

Intrauterine Pressure Catheter

- Quantitative measurement of uterine contraction frequency, duration, intensity and resting tone
- Three types:
  - Fluid-filled
  - Transducer-tipped
  - Air-coupled or sensor-tipped

© 2010 AWHONN 157

Benefits of Intrauterine Pressure Catheter (IUPC)

- Accurate assessment of frequency, duration, intensity of contractions and resting tone
- Withdrawal of amniotic fluid for testing
- Amnioinfusion port
- May be recalibrated or flushed to validate accuracy of internal monitoring

© 2010 AWHONN 158

CAT III

Pat (cont.)

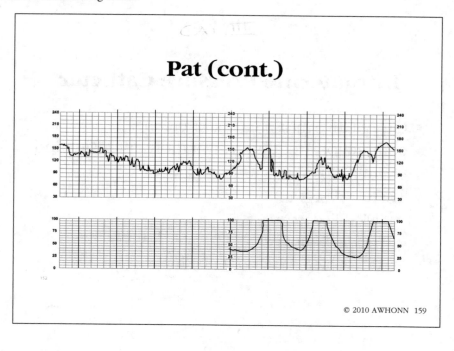

© 2010 AWHONN 159

CAT III

Pat (cont.)

ABSENT
VARIABILITY

not modera

at least
3-6 cycle
un 1 min pe
MODERATE
6-25

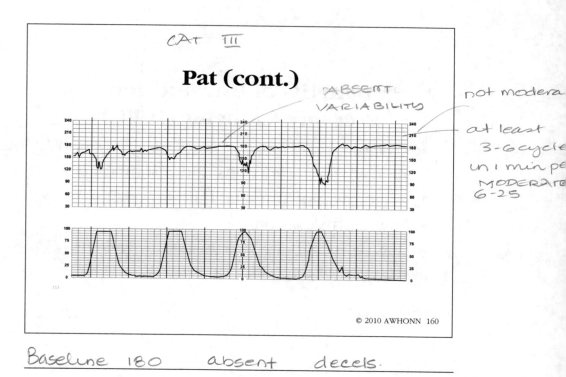

© 2010 AWHONN 160

Baseline 180   absent   decels.

Pat (cont.): Outcome

- Cesarean birth
- Male infant
- Apgar scores of 8/9
- Birth weight: 3.04 lb (1,380 g)
- IUGR
- 10% abruption

© 2010 AWHONN 161

Nicole, 27 Years Old
G_1, P_0, 39 Weeks' Gestation

- History: unremarkable
- Current pregnancy:
  - Serial ultrasounds at 18, 30, 34 and 36 weeks
  - Asymmetrical IUGR   THINK   after or fetus had insult that prevented some of its growth
  - Vaginal exam: 3 cm/90%/0   e.g. lower extremities but not brain

© 2010 AWHONN 162

symmetrical IUGR suggest 1st trimester insult affected entire fetus ∴ neurological damage.

Nicole (cont.): Admission Tracing

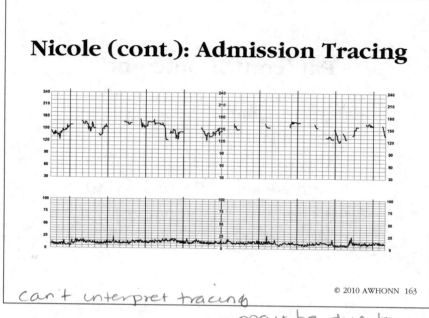

© 2010 AWHONN 163

Can't interpret tracing

OPTIONS place FSE; may be due to: maternal size,
↑ fetal movement

Troubleshooting the Ultrasound

- Confirm fetal position by Leopold's maneuvers
- Auscultate the FHR
- Reapply the monitor gel
- Reposition the transducer to detect fetal cardiac motion
- Reposition the mother
- Use real-time ultrasound visualization *to visualize fetus*
- Apply fetal spiral electrode (FSE)

© 2010 AWHONN 164

Troubleshooting
the Tocodynamometer

- Palpate for the point of strongest fundal intensity
- Place the toco flat and firm against the abdomen
- Check the monitor equipment
- Consider intrauterine pressure catheter monitoring

© 2010 AWHONN 165

Nicole (cont.)

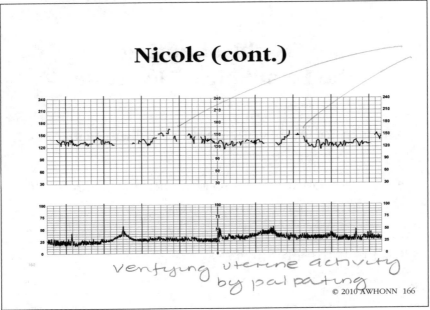

accels.

gaps in not a continuous 2 min period.

verifying uterine activity by palpating

© 2010 AWHONN 166

Baseline 130

Nicole (cont.)

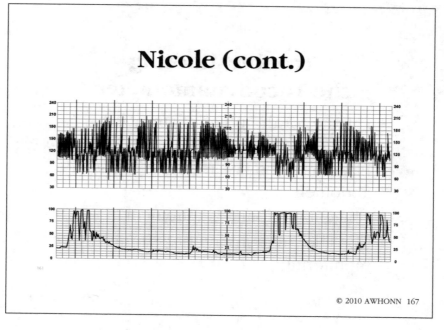

© 2010 AWHONN 167

Can't give a baseline ∴ go back to
previous 10 min to determine baseline
∴ troubleshoot by listening & counting
beats, US to verify

Troubleshooting
the Fetal Spiral Electrode

- Listen to what your ears are telling you

- Check connections to the monitor, electrode cable and presenting part

- Check the circuitry

© 2010 AWHONN 168

Troubleshooting
the Fetal Spiral Electrode (cont.)

- Check the on/off position of logic or electrocardiogram (ECG) disable switch
- Confirm the maternal pulse
- Auscultate with fetoscope to confirm the FHR
- Change the FSE

© 2010 AWHONN 169

Nicole (cont.): FSE, IUPC

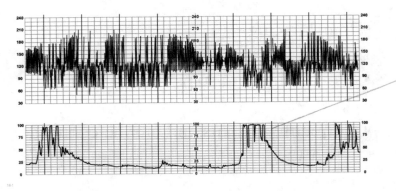

© 2010 AWHONN 170

seen in 2nd
stage of la

coughing,
pushing, vomiting

IUPC
indicates
picking up ctx

no improvement

Troubleshooting the IUPC

- Verify IUPC position (check markings at perineum and ask the patient to cough)
- Flush the catheter (if applicable)
- Recalibrate if:
  Resting tone = 25 mm/Hg
  - Resting tone is too high/too low despite palpation of soft uterus.
  - No contraction pattern exists with palpable contractions.
  - Artifact is present.
- Check the monitor for loose connections or re-zero the IUPC as needed
- Run the monitor's self-test feature

© 2010 AWHONN 171

Documentation

- Initial tracing

- Troubleshooting steps

- Current fetal status and uterine contraction pattern

© 2010 AWHONN 172

Nicole (cont.): Outcome

- Spontaneous vaginal birth
- Female infant
- Apgar scores of 8/9
- 5 lb, 7 oz (2,466 g)
- Cord blood pH 7.23, 7.26, arterial and venous, respectively
- Normal heart rhythm at 1 hour of age
- Home with mother

reflection of O₂ status of fetus in utero.

tells about maternal status

© 2010 AWHONN 173

Care and Storage of Equipment

- Handle with caution due to fragile nature
- Never immerse transducers or cables in water, unless indicated by manufacturer
- Clean monitor, transducers and cables with approved disinfectant
- Loosely coil cables for storage
- Don't force insertion of cables into monitor if they don't fit
- Dispose of or wash fetal monitor straps according to facility or manufacturers' recommendations

© 2010 AWHONN 174

Techniques Summary

- Methods for assessing FHR
- Methods for assessing uterine contractions
- Troubleshooting monitor information
- Decisions regarding methods of monitoring based on clinical situation

fetoscope
EFM
FSE
IUPC
PALPATION

© 2010 AWHONN 175

Choosing Physiologically Based Interventions

© 2010 AWHONN 176

Physiologic Goals

- Support maternal coping and labor progress
- Maximize uterine blood flow c̄ wedge
- Maximize umbilical circulation
- Maximize oxygenation △ position, if tachysystole tx c̄ terb
- Maintain appropriate uterine activity palpate or IUPC

© 2010 AWHONN 177

AFTER EPIDURAL
- place pt on side
(NOT FLAT ON BACK

Interventions to Support
Coping and Labor Progress:
Setting the Stage for Positive Coping

- Review plans/expectations with the woman and her partner, friends or family
- Maintain calm environment whenever possible
- Include family members where appropriate

© 2010 AWHONN 178

Interventions to Support Coping and Labor Progress: Judicious Use of Technology

- Stay at the bedside as much as possible
- Assess patient needs when selecting a monitoring method
- Use frequent position changes and upright positioning
- Minimize use of technology and avoid unnecessary intervention when possible

© 2010 AWHONN 179

Determining Interventions and Goals

- Cervical exam
- Review of uterine activity and palpation of tone
- Evaluation of maternal vital signs
- Assessment of unit resources/workload

© 2010 AWHONN 180

Interventions to Maximize Uterine Blood Flow

- Anxiety/pain reduction

- Maternal position change

- Hydration ⟹ ↓ ctx

- Medication (terbutaline)

© 2010 AWHONN 181

Maternal Catecholamine Release

| Maternal pain/anxiety | → | Catecholamine release | → | Shunting of maternal blood flow toward vital organs |

= SALVAGE to heart, brain adrenals.

| Blood shunted away from uterus | → | Less blood flow to intervillous space and uterine cells | → | Depleted oxygenation of fetus; less effective uterine activity |

© 2010 AWHONN 182

Interventions to Maximize Umbilical Circulation

- Maternal position change

- Elevation of presenting part

- Amnioinfusion

© 2010 AWHONN 183

oligohydramnios, variables, (arm resting on cord) cord compression
prolapse cord = umbilical cord is out of cervix
∴ no blood flow

Interventions to Maximize Oxygenation

- Maternal position change
- Maternal hydration
- Maternal breathing techniques
- Maternal supplemental oxygen (do not give O_2 if not needed)
- Correct or treat underlying disease
  e.g. DIABETES if hypoglycemia can have absent variability

© 2010 AWHONN 184

JAMA

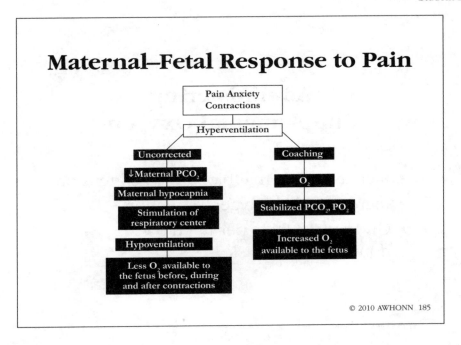

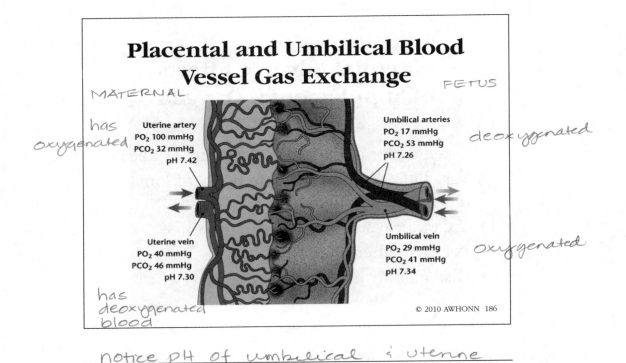

MATERNAL

FETUS

has oxygenated

deoxygenated

has deoxygenated blood

oxygenated

notice pH of umbilical & uterine artery & veins

Administering Supplemental Oxygen

- Increases maternal blood oxygen tension
- Increases fetal oxygen saturation
- Given at 10 liters per minute via nonrebreather mask

© 2010 AWHONN 187

Potential Adverse Effects of Supplemental Oxygen

hyperoxia → hypoxia

- Potential for creation of oxygen-free radicals
  => damage cellular membrane structures & DNA.
- Very little data available on effect of long-term administration
- Try other resuscitative techniques first
- Remove other sources of stress
- Discontinue as soon as possible

© 2010 AWHONN 188

If TACHYSYSTOLE
- stop pitocin
- ∆ position
- hydration
* then oxygen*

discontinue O2 once FHR recovers.

Interventions
to Modify Uterine Activity

- Maternal position change *[handwritten: if on back UA will be ↑ lateral position best]*
- Appropriate use of uterotonic drugs
- Hydration
- Tocolytic medication
- Appropriate second stage of labor care

© 2010 AWHONN 189

Physiology of Prolonged Valsalva *[handwritten: i.e. pushing]*

Long valsalva maneuver → ↑ Abdominal and intrathoracic pressure →

↑ Vasoconstriction / ↓ Cardiac output → Maternal blood flow ↓ →

↑ Intrauterine pressure → Uterine blood flow ↓ →

Blood flow in the intervillous space ↓

Blood flow in the intervillous space ↓ → ↓ pH, pO$_2$ base excess / ↑ pCO$_2$ nonreassuring FHR → ↑ Newborn acidemia / ↓ Apgar scores

(Adapted from Barnett, M. M., & Humenick S. S. (1982). Infant outcome in relation to second stage labor pushing method. *Birth. 9*, 221–229).

© 2010 AWHONN 190

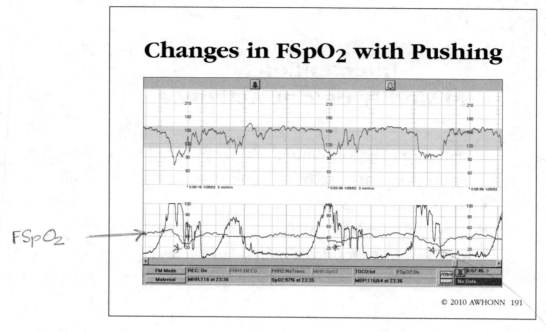

FSpO₂

avg. fetal O₂sat = 40-45% ; changes c̄ ctx.
allow the pt to rest between ctx

The Second Stage of Labor

- Two phases:
  - Initial latent phase
  - Active pushing phase
- Wait until the urge to push occurs before assisting with pushing efforts.
- Take advantage of the latent phase to let the fetus descend and the mother rest.

© 2010 AWHONN 192

Support Rather than Direct

- Support involuntary pushing:
  - Delay pushing until the urge to push is felt.
  - Coach only if guidance is needed.
- If direction and guidance are needed:
  - Discourage prolonged breath holding.
  - Discourage more than three pushing efforts.
  - Limit pushing efforts to 6–8 seconds each.
  - Do not discourage vocalization.

© 2010 AWHONN 193

Supporting the Fetus in the Active Phase of the Second Stage

- Take steps to maintain a normal FHR pattern while pushing
- Push with every other or every third contraction if necessary to help avoid recurrent FHR decelerations
- Reposition frequently to promote progress
- Use intrauterine resuscitation techniques when needed
- Avoid uterine tachysystole
- Avoid closed-glottis, valsalva pushing

© 2010 AWHONN 194

Betty, 33 Years Old
G_2, P_{1001}, 39 Weeks' Gestation

- Presented with vaginal bleeding
- Complained of decreased fetal movement
- Ultrasound done; placenta previa ruled out
- Vaginal exam: 3 cm/80%/-2 and cephalic presentation
- AROM—Large amount of thin green fluid
- FSE and IUPC applied

© 2010 AWHONN 195

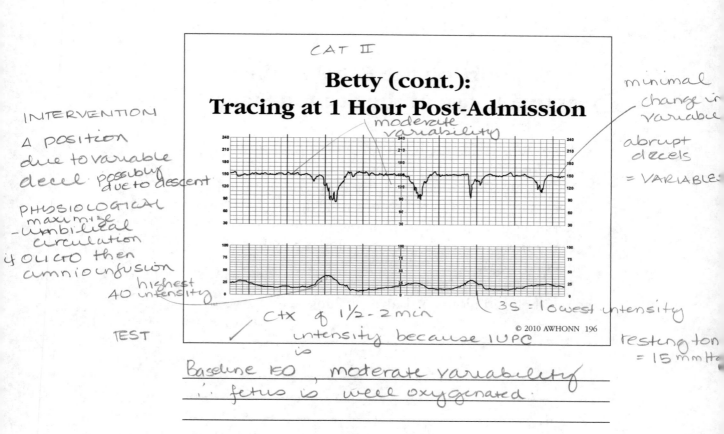

CAT II

Betty (cont.):
Tracing at 1 Hour Post-Admission

© 2010 AWHONN 196

Handwritten annotations:

INTERVENTION

A position due to variable decel possibly due to descent

PHYSIOLOGICAL — maximize umbilical circulation — if OLIGO then amnioinfusion

highest 40 intensity

TEST

moderate variability

minimal change in variable abrupt decels = VARIABLE

35 = lowest intensity

resting ton = 15 mmHg

Ctx of 1½-2 min intensity because IUPC is

Baseline 150, moderate variability ∴ fetus is well oxygenated.

Interventions

- Change maternal position
- Perform vaginal examination as indicated
- Palpate contractions and assess uterine tone
- Recheck maternal vital signs *to R/o chorio*
- Inform/support woman and her family
- Confer with Betty's other providers (CNM/MD)

© 2010 AWHONN 197

give O₂ because becoming recurrent variables

Betty (cont.): Outcome

- Vaginal delivery
- Apgar scores 5/8
- Nuchal cord ×3
- True knot in the cord
- 20% abruption
- Mild respiratory acidosis noted with arterial cord blood gases

© 2010 AWHONN 198

True Knot in Cord

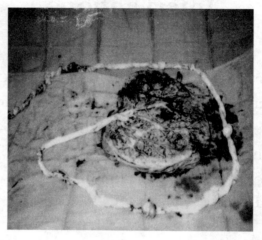

© 2010 AWHONN 199

Cord Entanglement

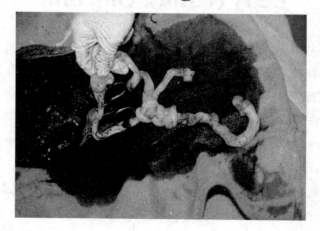

© 2010 AWHONN 200

Amnioinfusion

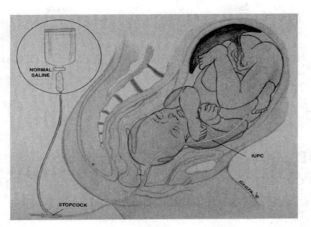

© 2010 AWHONN 201

Marsha, 20 Years Old
G_2, P_{1001}, 39 Weeks' Gestation

- History: unremarkable
- Current pregnancy:
  - No risk factors
  - Admitted in early labor
  - Vaginal exam: 2 cm/80%/-1; <u>spontaneous</u> *may see variables.*
    <u>rupture of membranes,</u> clear fluid, no odor
  - FHR 125, moderate variability, no decelerations
  - Uterine contractions every 3 min × 60–70 sec, moderate by palpation

© 2010 AWHONN 202

Marsha (cont.)

- Regional anesthesia at 11:45 (sitting position)

- Vital signs: BP 100/58, P 98, T 98.6°F (37°C)

- FHR 125 bpm, moderate variability, accelerations present, no decelerations prior to epidural administration

© 2010 AWHONN 203

Marsha (cont.): 15 Minutes Later

AFTER EPIDURAL.

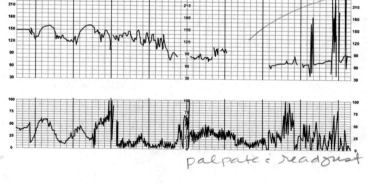

prolonged

palpate & readjust

© 2010 AWHONN 204

Can't interpret baseline there is no 2 min MARKED variability immediate intervention A position, SVE for cord prolapse notify primary provider, palpate uterus, hydrate, O₂. get OR ready.

Profound Drop in FHR: Immediate Interventions

- Call for help and notify primary care provider
- Perform vaginal exam
- Prepare to expedite birth
- Initiate intrauterine resuscitation:
    - Change maternal position and palpate uterus
    - Assess BP: medicate as indicated/ordered
    - Hydrate / iv fluids
    - Oxygenate

© 2010 AWHONN 205

_____

_____

_____

_____

Relaxation of the Uterus with Medications

- Tocolytic administration:

    - Enhance fetal oxygenation

    - Promote uterine relaxation

    - Increase uteroplacental blood flow

© 2010 AWHONN 206

_____

_____

_____

_____

Marsha (cont.)

Significant physiology:

- Hypotension?
- Compression of umbilical cord?
- Excessive uterine activity?
- Abruption?
- Sudden descent?

© 2010 AWHONN 207

ARTIFACT

Marsha (cont.)

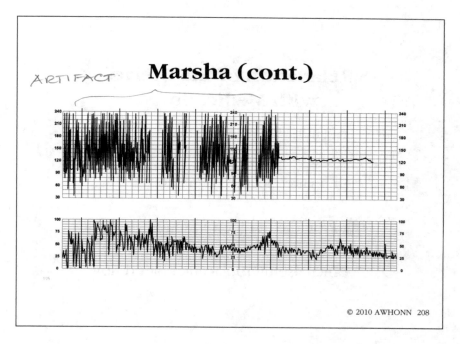

© 2010 AWHONN 208

Variability recovered not marked.
returned

READ CH ON

FETAL ACID BASE

Assessment
of Fetal Acid–Base Status

- Indirect methods:
  (not when fetus has a decel)
  - Fetal scalp stimulation   done when FHR is at baseline
  - Vibroacoustic stimulation/noise
  - Fetal pulse oximetry
- Direct methods:
  - Fetal scalp sampling
  - Umbilical cord blood sampling

© 2010 AWHONN 209

Fetal Scalp Stimulation Example

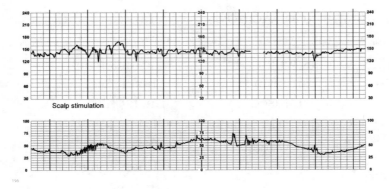

Scalp stimulation

© 2010 AWHONN 210

MODERATE VARIABILITY.

Fetal Scalp Sampling

- To perform, obtain a sample of fetal capillary blood from the fetal scalp.
- Many factors potentially affected results of the sample.
- It is rarely used in the United States today.
- Research involving fetal accelerations relating to a normal acid–base balance resulted from fetal scalp sampling.

© 2010 AWHONN 211

Umbilical Cord Blood Acid–Base Analysis

Respiratory Acidosis	Metabolic Acidosis
- $\uparrow CO_2$ levels	- $\uparrow$ lactic acid levels
- Occurs when fetal CO_2 cannot be easily diffused	- Results from anaerobic metabolism
- Can develop rapidly	- Takes longer to develop
- Can be corrected rapidly	- Takes longer to resolve

© 2010 AWHONN 212

ACIDOSIS

RESPIRATORY = occlusion of umbilical vein ⇒ build up of CO_2. ACUTE PROCESS - can be resolved quickly

METABOLIC = build up of lactic acid.
EVOLVES OVER TIME ∴ takes a longer time to resolve

lactic acid + O_2 → CO_2 + H_2O → excreted

Single-Digit Value Guideline
Initial Assessment of Umbilical Cord Blood Acid–Base Values

	Target Values	Metabolic Acidemia	Respiratory Acidemia
pH	≥ 7.10	< 7.10	< 7.10
pO_2 (mmHg)	> 20	< 20	variable
pCO_2 (mmHg)	< 60	< 60	> 60
Bicarbonate (mEq/L)	> 22	< 22	≥ 22
BD (mEq/L)	≤ 12	> 12	< 12
BE (mEq/L)	≥ -12	< -12	> -12

© 2010 AWHONN 213

BASE EXCESS measuring metabolic alkalosis expressed amt of acid/alkali to titrate pH of blood. BASE DEFICIT measuring metabolic acidosis.

Types of Acidosis

	pH	pCO_2	pO_2	BD
Respiratory	↓	↑	Variable	WNL
Metabolic	↓	WNL	↓	↑
Mixed	↓	↑	↓	↑

© 2010 AWHONN 214

Umbilical Arterial Cord Gas Values

Case #1

- pH = 7.22
- pO_2 = 28
- pCO_2 = 42
- Bicarbonate = 27
- BE = –6

NORMAL

Case #2

- pH = 7.02
- pO_2 = 19
- pCO_2 = 72
- Bicarbonate = 23
- BD = 10

RESPIRATORY ACEDEMIA.

© 2010 AWHONN 215

Vera, 32 Years Old
G_4, P_{2012}, 36 Weeks' Gestation

- History: unremarkable
- Current pregnancy:
  - Chicken pox at 6–8 weeks' gestation *early insuer to fetus*
  - Ultrasound at 32 and 35 weeks' gestation with body in < 10th, and BPD in 28th percentile
  - Current pregnancy history otherwise unremarkable
  - Admitted for labor induction IUGR

© 2010 AWHONN 216

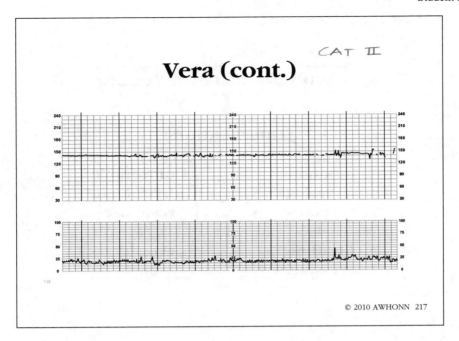

Vera (cont.)

CAT II

© 2010 AWHONN 217

Baseline 140   Variability - minimal
∅ accels, ∅ decels
Uterine activity - need to palpate &
            readjust toco.

When pt presents c̄ MINIMAL VARIABILITY.
 - assume progression of an insult

Interventions:
Minimal Variability on Admission

- Change maternal position
- Ask ᴍᴏᴍ about change in fetal movement
- Attempt to stimulate an acceleration
- Hydrate
- Consider oxygen administration
- Call for bedside evaluation

© 2010 AWHONN 218

maximize fetal blood flow.
oxygenate fetus

MINIMAL   - by itself does not predict
VARIABILITY   acidemia

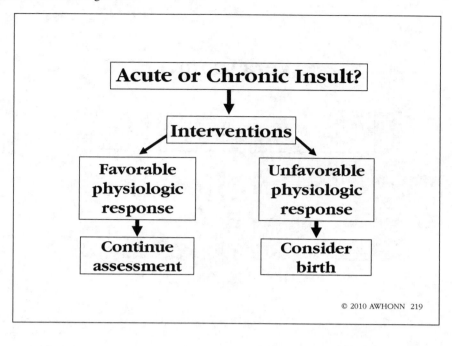

© 2010 AWHONN 219

INDUCTION WAS STARTED.

CAT III

ABSENT VARIABILITY

c̄ LATE DECELS

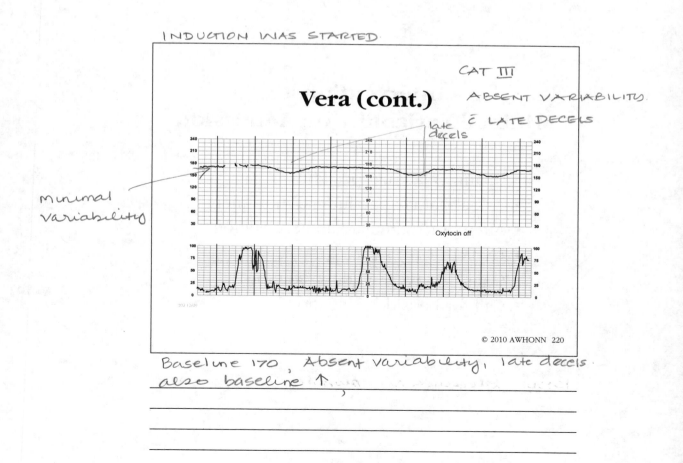

Vera (cont.)

late decels

minimal Variability

Oxytocin off

© 2010 AWHONN 220

Baseline 170, Absent variability, late decels.
also baseline ↑

Vera (cont.): Outcome

- Emergent cesarean birth
- Infant boy weighing 4 lb, 9 oz (2,070 g)
- Baby initially vigorous
- Apgar scores of 8/9
- Infant assessment at birth reveals multiple chicken pox scars on trunk and extremities
- Transferred to a tertiary care center
- Neurologic deficit was diagnosed after transfer

© 2010 AWHONN 221

Vera (cont.)

Arterial Cord Blood Gas Results
- pH   7.32
- pCO$_2$ 44.1
- pO$_2$ 20.2
- Bicarbonate   22.0
- Base deficit (BD)   3.7

© 2010 AWHONN 222

Fetus adequately oxygenated immediately prior to birth

Elizabeth, 36 Years Old
G_2, P_{0010}, 41 Weeks' Gestation

History:

- Spontaneous abortion at 10 weeks' gestation
- Admitted with spontaneous rupture of membranes × 12 hours, clear fluid, no odor
- Occasional uterine contractions, mild by palpation

© 2010 AWHONN 223

RISK FACTORS.

Elizabeth (cont.)

palpate ; adjust toco

© 2010 AWHONN 224

moderate variability , accels

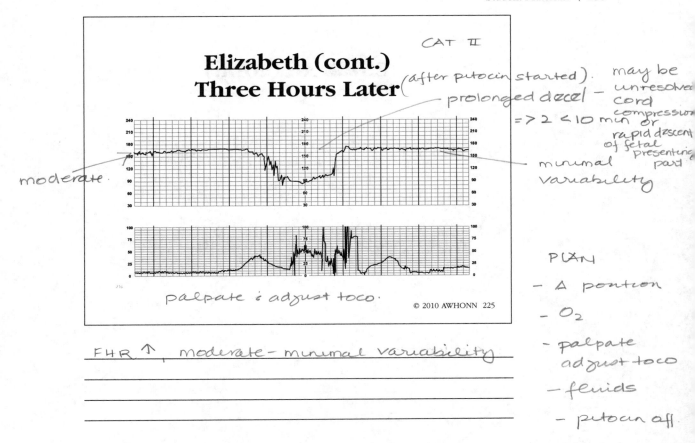

Elizabeth (cont.)
Three Hours Later

CAT II

(after pitocin started).

prolonged decel — *=> 2 < 10 min*

may be unresolved cord compression or rapid descent of fetal presenting part

moderate.

minimal variability

palpate & adjust toco.

© 2010 AWHONN 225

FHR ↑, moderate – minimal variability

PLAN
- Δ position
- O_2
- palpate adjust toco
- fluids
- pitocin off.

Elizabeth (cont.)

Goals:
- Maintain appropriate uterine activity *(turn pitocin off)*
- Maximize uterine blood flow *(hydration)*
- Maximize umbilical circulation *(Δ position)*
- Maximize oxygenation

© 2010 AWHONN 226

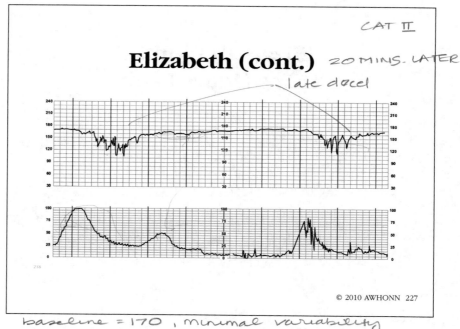

CAT II

Elizabeth (cont.) 20 MINS. LATER

late decel

© 2010 AWHONN 227

to determine
Δ in baseline —

baseline = 170, minimal variability
elevated baseline = TACHYCARDIA
has to be for at least 10 mins

palpate & adjust toco, hydrate, O₂
temp check (possible chorio) tylenol

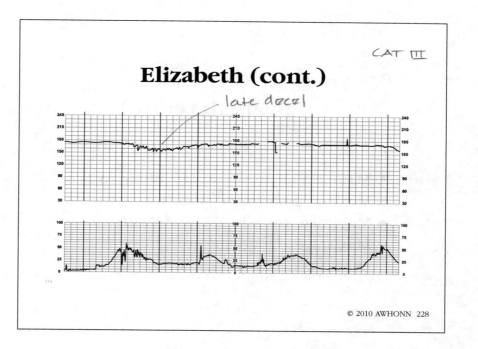

CAT III

Elizabeth (cont.)

late decel

© 2010 AWHONN 228

ABSENT variability & elevated
baseline & late decel.

Elizabeth (cont.): Outcome
Fetal Arterial Cord Blood Values

- pH ↓   7.09
- pCO_2 ↑   80 mmHg
- pO_2 18 mmHg
- BD ↑   15 mEq/L

© 2010 AWHONN 229

MIXED ACIDOSIS

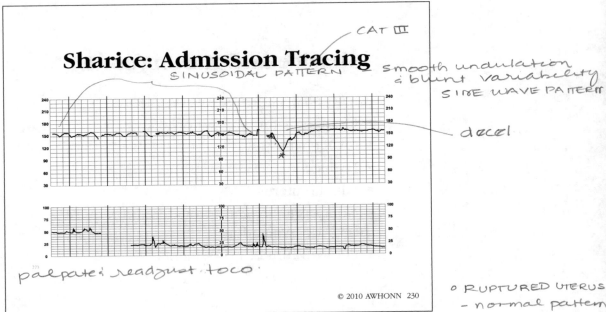

CAT III

Sharice: Admission Tracing

SINUSOIDAL PATTERN

smooth undulation
& blunt variability
SINE WAVE PATTERN

decel

palpate & readjust toco

© 2010 AWHONN 230

° RUPTURED UTERUS
   - normal pattern
     to no activity

° SINUSOIDAL can be due to.
- bleeding abruption, fetal anemia, hypoxemia
opiates, anencephalic fetus
A position, hydrate, notify MD

° IF ABRUPTION
- high frequency low volume uterine activity (ie. a lot of ctx
           & low waves

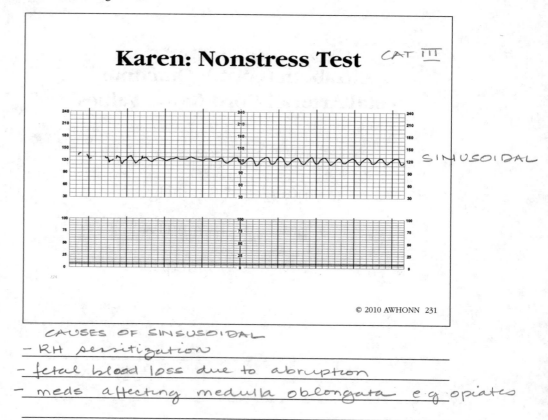

Karen: Nonstress Test CAT III

SINUSOIDAL

© 2010 AWHONN 231

CAUSES OF SINUSOIDAL
- RH sensitization
- fetal blood loss due to abruption
- meds affecting medulla oblongata e.g. opiates

Sharice and Karen (cont.)

Rapid assessments/interventions:
- Change maternal position
- Oxygenate
- Hydrate
- Palpate uterus
- Notify primary care provider and request bedside evaluation
- Perform further assessment

© 2010 AWHONN 232

Sharice, 23 Years Old
G_1, P_0, 33 Weeks Gestation

Current pregnancy:
- Complaint of decreased fetal movement
- BPP 2/10: =

0-2 - Amniotic fluid volume (2) *points*

0-2 - Absent fetal breathing movement (0)

0-2 - Absent fetal movement (0)

0-2 - Absent fetal tone (0)

0-2 - Nonreactive nonstress test (0)

© 2010 AWHONN 233

Sharice (cont.)

Current pregnancy:
- Cesarean birth
- Baby's Apgar scores of 2/5/7 at 1, 5 and 10 minutes, respectively
- Baby very pale with suspected fetal–maternal hemorrhage, unknown source
- Placenta normal: no abruption

placenta pale = placenta not well perfused
placenta yellow = infection

© 2010 AWHONN 234

Baby's hct is higher than maternal can be high as 61 ±7 acceptable. Normal Hg = 19 physiological jaundice quick breakdown of RBC. which the liver can't handle.

Karen, 26 Years Old
G_4, P_{3003}, 37 Weeks Gestation

Current pregnancy:
- Complaint of decreased fetal movement
- Ultrasound examination revealed anencephaly

© 2010 AWHONN 235

Clinical Decision Making

- Maternal–fetal physiology
- Physical assessment
- Patient interview
- Technology capabilities
- Core knowledge
- Communication
- Documentation

© 2010 AWHONN 236

Collaborative Model

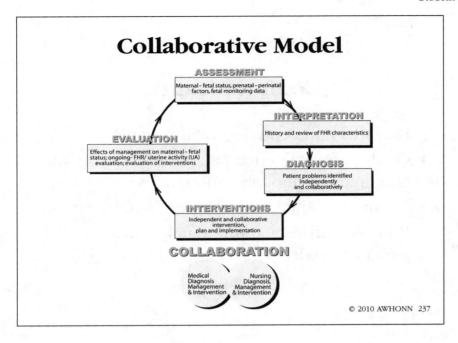

ASSESSMENT
Maternal – fetal status, prenatal – perinatal factors, fetal monitoring data

INTERPRETATION
History and review of FHR characteristics

EVALUATION
Effects of management on maternal – fetal status; ongoing- FHR/ uterine activity (UA) evaluation; evaluation of interventions

DIAGNOSIS
Patient problems identified independently and collaboratively

INTERVENTIONS
Independent and collaborative intervention, plan and implementation

COLLABORATION

Medical Diagnosis Management & Intervention

Nursing Diagnosis, Management & Intervention

© 2010 AWHONN 237

Communication and Accountability

© 2010 AWHONN 238

Communication

- Essential and central to quality care
- Quality can influence patient safety, care and outcomes for mothers and babies
- Channels should remain open in all directions
- Primary purpose: **appropriately meet patient's needs**

© 2010 AWHONN 239

Communication (cont.)

- All providers on the perinatal team make important contributions.

- The patient is the center of communication and care.

- Patients' input should be encouraged and valued.

© 2010 AWHONN 240

Communication (cont.)

- Effective, patient-centered communication can contribute to a reduction in medical–legal exposure.

- Providing safe, quality care is one component of protection against legal liability.

© 2010 AWHONN 241

Essential Principles of Effective Teamwork

- Teams, rather than individuals, create optimal performance.
- Each team member is valued for his or her unique experience, knowledge and contributions.
- Professionals are responsible and accountable for their individual behavior.
- Effective teams work collectively to achieve an agreed-upon goal: to achieve the best possible outcome.

© 2010 AWHONN 242

Communication and FHM

- Communication issues are the leading root cause for sentinel events in the intrapartum setting.
- Common terminology for all team members:
  - AWHONN and ACOG recommend 2008 NICHD guidelines.
- Goal of bedside clinician is to communicate a clear picture of the clinical situation.

© 2010 AWHONN 243

Essential Principles
of Effective Communication

Open   Clear   Honest

Concise   Timely   Respectful

Be Direct:
When you know what you need,
ask for it!

© 2010 AWHONN 244

Being Direct

- What is happening
- Assessment of situation
- Recommendations for care
- Urgency with which action is needed

➡ Synthesis of information is essential
- Confirm mutual understanding

© 2010 AWHONN 245

Briefings and Assertion

SBAR:

- Situation
- Background
- Assessment
- *Recommendation*

(Preston, P. [2004]. Practical perinatal safety: Some
high yield interventions. Antepartum & Intrapartum
Management Conference, San Francisco, CA, June 19, 2004.)

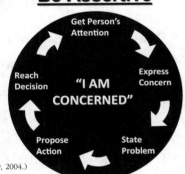

Be Assertive

(Simpson & Knox [2003], *AWHONN Lifelines)*

© 2010 AWHONN 246

CHAT as a Communication Method

- CHAT:
  - Context
  - History
  - Assessment
  - Tentative plan

© 2010 AWHONN 247

Structured Formats for Communication

- These are universal tools for ALL clinicians.
- Expectations for providing and receiving information are clear to all team members.
- Communications regarding emergent situations require special considerations.
- Clear expectations for actions are given before communication is terminated.

© 2010 AWHONN 248

Communication Examples

- **Situation:** I'm calling about Ashley Stewart in Room 10. She is now completely dilated and 0 station. She has had intermittent variable decelerations for the past 20 minutes. The FHR baseline is 140 bpm and there is moderate variability.

© 2010 AWHONN 249

UNCLEAR PICTURE

did not give G P, OB Hx & Med Hx, Membrane status, is PEDS needed, ctx ·

Communication Examples (cont.)

- **Background:** The patient is a G_4, P_{3003} at 38 1/7 weeks who was admitted 5 hours ago with SROM, clear fluid. The variable decelerations have not resolved with position changes or fluid bolus.

→ INTERVENTION

© 2010 AWHONN 250

UNCLEAR PICTURE

SROM no vsigns given, length of time for variable decels not given

Communication Examples (cont.)

PRECIPITOUS LABOR

- **Assessment:** Ashley dilated from 5 to 10 cm over the last 30 minutes.
- **Recommendation:** Birth is imminent. I need you to come now. When can I expect to see you?

© 2010 AWHONN 251

Communication Example (cont.)

"I wanted to let you know that I discontinued the oxytocin infusion because of tachysystole. I also gave an IV fluid bolus of 500 mL of lactated *(@ what* Ringer's solution and assisted the patient to a lateral position to decrease uterine activity. The FHR tracing is normal. As soon as the uterine activity returns to normal, I'll restart the oxytocin. Do you want me to call back in an hour with a status report?" *don't ask for permission.*

© 2010 AWHONN 252

o FHR
- baseline
- variability
- accels, decels
- monitor ↗ external
    ↘ internal
  MONITOR MODE / IUPC

o CTX ↘ TOCO
- frequency.
- duration
- palpation
- uterine resting tone
- MONITOR MODE ↗ TOCO
    ↘ IUPC

Communication Example (cont.)

e.g. of DIRECT COMMUNICATION.

"I am concerned about your order to start oxytocin induction on Ms. Lee when the FHR pattern shows minimal variability without accelerations after scalp stimulation. I am going to wait to begin the oxytocin until you are able to come in and see the patient. I want us to review the tracing together. When can I expect to see you?"

© 2010 AWHONN 253

Communicating Urgency

"I'm calling about Ms. Garcia, the patient we spoke about earlier. The FHR has a prolonged deceleration in the 90s for 5 minutes that has not resolved with interventions. I need you here now. When can I expect to see you?"

© 2010 AWHONN 254

Communication Clarity

"My patient's tracing doesn't look good. She's having some contractions now, but it is flat and there are some decels. What do you want to do?"

© 2010 AWHONN 255

Pt's identity unclear, did not indicate type of decels, do not say "flat" use correct terminology

---

Clarity, Urgency and Expected Action

CNM to MD

- This is Sally Smith. I'm the CNM on-call in L&D.
- One of our patients presented with 10 cm blood clots on her underpads, abdominal pain and FHR baseline of 70 with absent variability. I need you here now. I think she is abrupting.
- When can I expect to see you?

© 2010 AWHONN 256

Pt's identity unclear, what type of decels, flat-

Responsiveness

- Physician's response:
  - To confirm, the patient is actively bleeding with suspected abruption and there is fetal bradycardia. Correct?
  - I'm at home. I'll be there in 10 minutes.
  - Initiate the emergency cesarean section protocol.

© 2010 AWHONN 257

Transfers of Care (Handoffs)

- Transfers of care are a time of vulnerability.
- Whenever possible:
  - Use face-to-face reporting
  - Assess patient status together
  - Solicit oncoming provider's questions and opinion
  - Provide written summary of critical information:
    - Use protocols or checklists to ensure completeness
    - Ensure information is up-to-date and accurate

© 2010 AWHONN 258

More Communication Strategies

- Closed loop

- Briefs

- Huddles

- Debrief

© 2010 AWHONN 259

_____

_____

_____

_____

Documentation

- Streamlined, factual and objective record of the care provided
- Contains *only* and *all* clinically relevant information
- Duplication of information should be avoided:
  - Whenever possible, avoid documenting routine care on the EFM tracing when it is also being recorded in the chart.
- Detailed descriptions of tracings are unnecessary

© 2010 AWHONN 260

_____

_____

_____

_____

Documentation (cont.)

- Reflects a systematic admission assessment and ongoing assessments of the laboring woman and fetus

- Includes assessments and documentation in time frames that are consistent with the patient's condition, as well as institutional and professional guidelines

- Reflects facility policies and procedures for assessment and documentation of maternal/fetal status

© 2010 AWHONN 261

Flow Sheet for FHR Documentation

Date of Record:					
	TIME				
Cervix	Dilation				
	Effacement				
	Station				
Fetal Heart	Baseline Rate				
	Variability				
	Accelerations				
	Decelerations				
	STIM/pH				
	Monitor Mode				
Uterine Activity	Frequency				
	Duration				
	Intensity				
	Resting Tone				
	Monitor Mode				
	Coping				
	Maternal Position				
	O_2: L/min/Mask				
	IV				
	Initials				

© 2010 AWHONN 262

Identifying Information on Tracing

- Patient name
- Hospital identification number
- Date and time monitoring began
- Mode of monitoring
- Calibration test, per facility protocol

© 2010 AWHONN 263

_____

_____

_____

_____

Questions Regarding Documenting EFM Assessments

- FHR information?

- Uterine activity information?

- Frequency of assessments?

- Frequency of documentation?

© 2010 AWHONN 264

_____

_____

_____

_____

Documentation of FHR Characteristics

Auscultation	Electronic Monitoring
Rate	Rate
Rhythm	Variability
Increases and decreases	Periodic and episodic changes
	Pattern evolution
Associated clinical findings	
Communications	

(handwritten notes):
regular
irregular

= decels, accels.
e.g. tachycardia
bradycardia

© 2010 AWHONN 265

Clarifying Confusing EFM Patterns

- Assessment of the baseline variability
- Evolution of the tracing—what was it when admitted and what is it now
- Other clinical indicators of fetal status and progress in labor
- Maternal–fetal response to interventions
- Categorization of tracing

© 2010 AWHONN 266

WHEN AMNIOINFUSION GIVEN:
- palpate uterus for resting tone.
- look in vagina for fluid coming out

Documenting Uterine Activity

Palpation	Tocodynamometer	Intrauterine Pressure Catheter
Frequency		
In minutes from beginning of one contraction to the beginning of the next		
Duration		
In seconds; average length of contractions		
Intensity		
Mild, moderate, strong	Mild, moderate, strong	mmHg _and_ palpation
Resting Tone		
Soft or firm	By palpation: soft, firm	mmHg _and_ palpation
Descriptive		
Degree of associated pain and maternal coping		
Normal uterine activity or _tachysystole_		

© 2010 AWHONN 267

---

accel
EPISODIC without ctx.

EFM Tracing Analysis #1

not a variable.

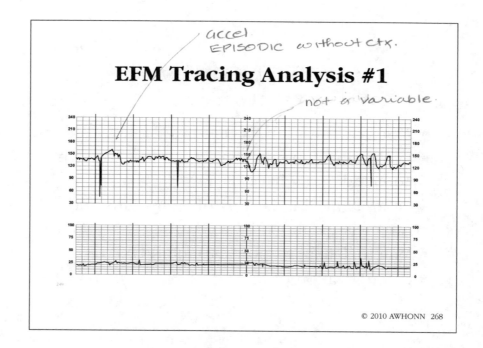

© 2010 AWHONN 268

135, moderate variability
PERIODIC CHANGES.

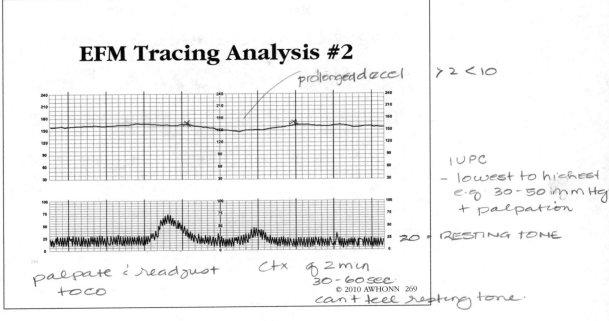

EFM Tracing Analysis #2

prolonged decel   >2 <10

IUPC
- lowest to highest
   e.g 30-50 mmHg
   + palpation

20 = RESTING TONE

palpate & readjust toco

Ctx q 2 min 30-60 sec.

© 2010 AWHONN 269

can't feel resting tone.

Baseline 160, variability absent

PERIODIC CHANGES - prolonged decel

palpation req'd for both toco & IUPC
   normal intensity 15-25 mm Hg
   bed needs to be at the same level of IUPC to get correct reading.

Frequency of Assessments and Documentation

- How often should maternal–fetal status be assessed?

- How often should maternal–fetal status be documented?

© 2010 AWHONN 270

Suggested Auscultation Frequency

	Latent Phase	Active First Stage	Active Second Stage
ACNM		Every 15–30 minutes	Every 5 minutes
AWHONN		Every 15–30 minutes	Every 5–15 minutes
ACOG, AAP		Every 15–30 minutes	Every 5 minutes
RCOG		Every 15 minutes	Every 5 minutes
SOGC	At the time of assessment and approximately every 1 hour	Every 15–30 minutes	Every 15 minutes then every 5 minutes after pushing initiated

(AAP & ACOG, 2007; ACNM, 2007; ACOG, 2005; AWHONN, 2009; Feinstein, Sprague, & Trepanier, 2008; RCOG, 2001; SOGC, 2007)

© 2010 AWHONN 271

[handwritten notes:]

consistent

ACTIVE FIRST STAGE ≥ 4 cm dilation & ctx q 2-3 for >

LATENT PHASE not in labor, not ctx consistently

Frequency of EFM Evaluations

AWHONN, 2009 AAP & ACOG, 2007	Active First Stage	Active Second Stage
Normal labor	Every 30 minutes	Every 15 minutes
Risk factors Present - Medical/OB risk - Oxytocin	Every 15 minutes	Every 5 minutes
SOGC, 2007	Active First Stage	Active Second Stage
All women receiving EFM	Every 15 minutes	Every 5 minutes

© 2010 AWHONN 272

Assessment vs. Documentation

Key Points:

- Assessments are conducted at intervals appropriate to the maternal–fetal condition.

- Documentation may not have to occur at the same intervals as assessment.

- Documentation should reflect a complete record of all assessments.

© 2010 AWHONN 273

Components of Fetal Monitoring Documentation

- Assessments
- Pertinent events and actions
- Clinical interventions
- Maternal–fetal responses to interventions
- Notification of primary care provider or other team members

© 2010 AWHONN 274

Documentation Example

- Repositioned to right side
- IV bolus of 500 mL LR
- O_2 at 10 L/min per nonrebreather face mask
- Maternal BP returned to 100/70 from 90/48
- Moderate variability, baseline 155 bpm following interventions
- Oxygen discontinued
- Dr. _____ notified of above findings.
  Signature

© 2010 AWHONN 275

Communication
Patient Teaching about FHM

- Inform mother and partner about the purpose and method of fetal monitoring.
- Discuss the FHR tracing and usual baseline rate.
- Discuss the uterine contraction tracing and the timing of contractions.
- Explain volume control.
- Explain positioning and the implications for ambulation as appropriate.
- Inform mother how to contact her nurse

© 2010 AWHONN 276

Dawn, 24 Years Old
G$_2$, P$_{1001}$, 38 3/7 Weeks Gestation

- History: unremarkable
- Current pregnancy:
  - Twins (dichorionic/diamniotic)
  - No other risk factors

© 2010 AWHONN 277

Dawn (cont.): Tracing of Twins

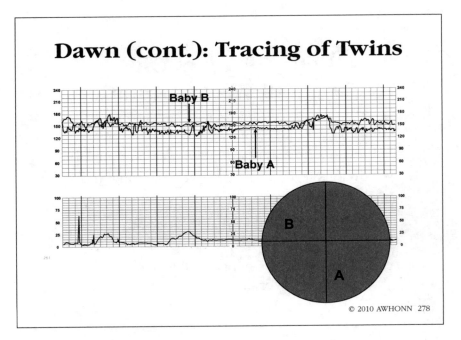

© 2010 AWHONN 278

BABY A   140 baseline, moderate, accels, & decels.
monitor mode   ctx q 2½ mins   duration 50-70

BABY B
adequate ctx q 2-3 mins

Dawn (cont.): Flow Sheet Documentation of Twins

Date of Record:	6/14/2009				
	TIME		1:00		
		:15			
Cervix	Dilation				
	Effacement				
	Station				
Fetal Heart	Baseline Rate	A 140 / B 155			
	Variability	A Mod / B Mod			
	Accelerations	+/+			
	Decelerations	none			
	STIM/pH				
	Monitor Mode	A FSE/B US			
Uterine Activity	Frequency	q 3-5			
	Duration	60–80 sec			
	Intensity	25–60 mmHg			
	Resting Tone	5–15 mmHg			
	Monitor Mode	IUPC			
	Coping	Well			
	Maternal Position	Rocking Chair			
	O₂: L/min/Mask				
	IV				
	Initials	NN			

Beth, 29 Years Old
G_3, P_{1101}, 38 Weeks Gestation

- History:
  - Previous preterm birth at 23 weeks, nonviable
  - Previous term birth at 39 weeks, living and well
- Current pregnancy:
  - No risk factors other than history of preterm labor
  - Reason for assessment: SROM; painful contractions every 2 minutes

Beth (cont.)

- Vital signs: Bp 126/68, P 78, R 18, T 98.2°F (36.7°C)
- Uterine contractions every 2 minutes; mild-strong by palpation
- Vaginal exam: 4 cm/80%/-1, vertex
- US and toco applied
- Beth is deep breathing to cope with contractions

© 2010 AWHONN 281

Beth (cont.): Admission Tracing

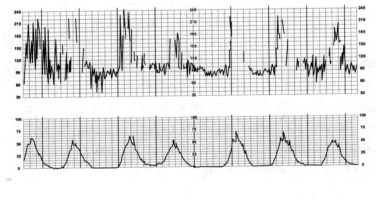

ALWAYS ASSESS MATERNAL PULSE

tachysystole

© 2010 AWHONN 282

Both FHR tracing & uterine activity need to be reassessed.

PLAN FIRST assess maternal pulse, US for cardiac activity ask pt about fetal movement,

Communication Nurse to Beth

- How will you talk with her?
- How will you answer her questions?
- What questions can you ask Beth in order to obtain more information?
- What will you document?

Beth (cont.)

Nurse to Physician/Midwife Reporting

"_____, this is Jeremy Jones, L&D nurse. I am calling to tell you that Beth, a gravida 3, para 1 with an uncomplicated history arrived here about 20 minutes ago. She is in early labor, but we have not been able to detect a fetal heart rate. The resident scanned her and was not able to visualize any cardiac activity."

Beth (cont.)

Nurse to Physician/Midwife Reporting (cont.)
"Beth is contracting every 1–3 minutes, lasting
50–120 seconds, with coupling. Contractions
palpate mild to moderate. She is dilated 4 cm, 80%
effaced, -1 station. She had spontaneous rupture
of membranes with scant fluid. She is really
worried about the status of the baby. I need to
have you come to the hospital right away."

[handwritten annotation: = twin ctx (not effective)]

© 2010 AWHONN 285

Beth (cont.)

Date of Record: 6/25/2008					
TIME			12:00		
		:15			
Cervix	Dilation	4			
	Effacement	80			
	Station	-1			
Fetal Heart	Baseline Rate	none			
	Variability	0			
	Accelerations	0			
	Decelerations	0			
	STIM/pH				
	Monitor Mode				
Uterine Activity	Frequency	q 2.5–3.5			
	Duration	50–120, coupling			
	Intensity	Mild-mod			
	Resting Tone	soft			
	Monitor Mode	Toco/palp			
	Coping	Anxious			
	Maternal Position	lateral			
	O₂: L/min/Mask				
	IV				
	Initials	SL			

© 2010 AWHONN 286

Beth (cont.): Documentation

Unable to differentiate MHR and FHR by auscultation. Toco and US applied. EFM shows irregular and bradycardic FHR pattern with frequent contractions. EFM volume increased, maternal brachial pulse palpated. HR on monitor synchronous with maternal pulse. Charge nurse and ____MD/CNM notified of inability to hear FHR and above findings. Beth very anxious, crying. Husband upset also but trying to comfort her. ____ on the way in to evaluate. – *J. Jones, RN*

Beth (cont.)

Nurse-to-Patient Communication

"Beth and Jeff, I just spoke with _____, and they are concerned for both of you. Dr/CNM wanted me to tell you that they will be here in 10 minutes."

Remember ...

Healthcare professionals should be familiar with current guidelines and recommendations relevant to their practice.

Examples:
- National (laws, regulations)
- State/provincial (statutes, nurse practice acts)
- Community standards
- Institutional (policies, procedures and protocols)
- Professional associations (practice guidelines)

© 2010 AWHONN 289

Conflict and Conflict Management

- Occasional conflict is a fact of professional life.
- Honest differences of opinion are to be expected.
- At times it may not be possible to resolve these conflicts in a time frame appropriate to the patient's condition.
- Chain of command/chain of authority is occasionally needed.

© 2010 AWHONN 290

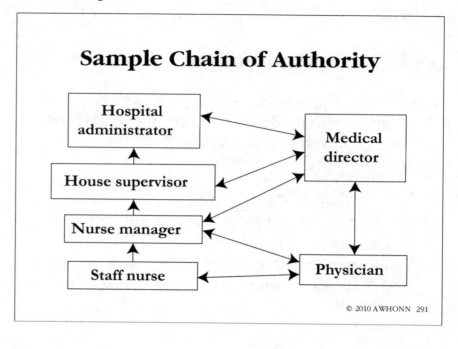

Sample Chain of Authority

Summary

- Collegial communication

- Documentation of care

Evaluation and Synthesis

© 2010 AWHONN   293

Synthesis

- Clear collaborative goals for care
- Physiology and historical data
- Selection/verification of assessment techniques and interventions
- Fetal heart/uterine contraction interpretation
- Timely and effective communication and teamwork

© 2010 AWHONN   294

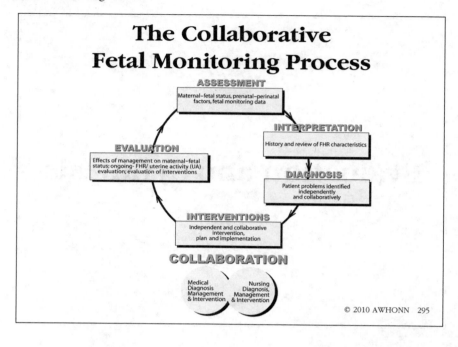

The Collaborative Fetal Monitoring Process

ASSESSMENT
Maternal–fetal status, prenatal–perinatal factors, fetal monitoring data

INTERPRETATION
History and review of FHR characteristics

DIAGNOSIS
Patient problems identified independently and collaboratively

INTERVENTIONS
Independent and collaborative intervention, plan and implementation

EVALUATION
Effects of management on maternal–fetal status; ongoing- FHR/ uterine activity (UA) evaluation; evaluation of interventions

COLLABORATION

Medical Diagnosis Management & Intervention

Nursing Diagnosis, Management & Intervention

© 2010 AWHONN   295

Pamela, 26 Years Old
G$_2$, P$_{1001}$, 39 Weeks Gestation

- History: unremarkable
- Current pregnancy:
  - Preeclampsia
  - BP 136/92–148/96
  - Sonograms times 2
  - Reactive NST times 3

© 2010 AWHONN   296

Pamela (cont.): Admission Assessment

- Admitted for induction of labor for preeclampsia
- Vaginal exam: 3 cm/50%/-2; cephalic
- Vital signs: BP 138/88, P 80, R 18, T 98.6°F (37°C)
- No contractions, intact membranes

© 2010 AWHONN   297

CAT I

Pamela (cont.): Admission Tracing (0800)

palpate & readjust toco

© 2010 AWHONN   298

Baseline 145   Variability moderate
c accels ø decels

Pamela (cont.): Risks for Decreased Uteroplacental Perfusion

can.

- Preeclampsia

- Oxytocin use

CAT I

Pamela (cont.): 1030 (2½ hours later)

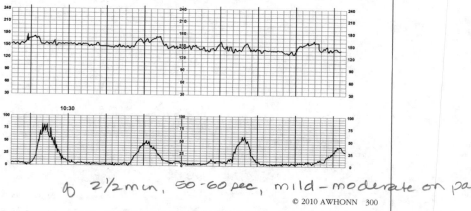

q 2½ min, 50-60 sec, mild-moderate on palpa

c̄ accels, ∅ decels.

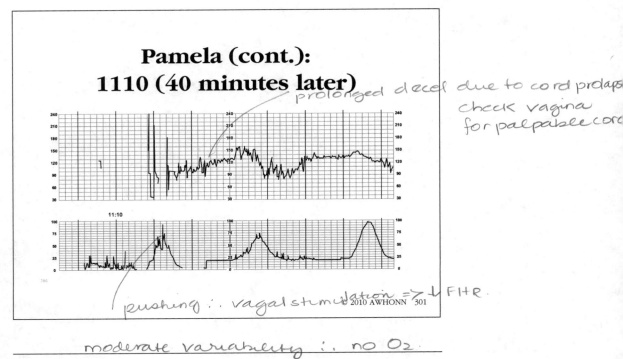

Pamela (cont.):
1110 (40 minutes later)

prolonged decel due to cord prolapse
check vagina
for palpable cord

pushing ∴ vagal stimulation ⇒ ↓ FHR

© 2010 AWHONN 301

moderate variability ∴ no O₂

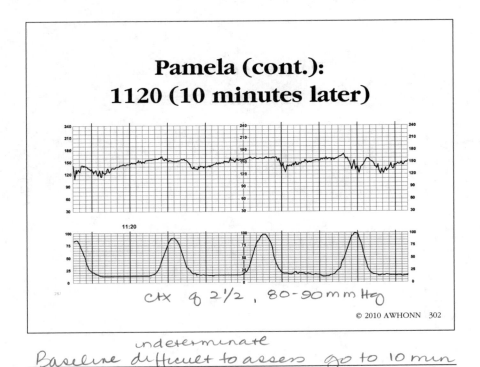

Pamela (cont.):
1120 (10 minutes later)

ctx q 2½, 80–90 mm Hg

© 2010 AWHONN 302

undeterminate
Baseline difficult to assess   go to 10 min
prior in tracing
Baseline 160, variability minimal
variable decels

ctx should not last longer than 1 min

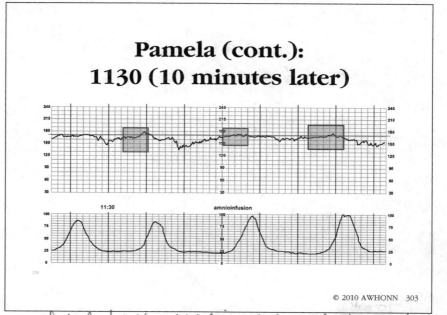

= fetal tachycardia sign of utero placental insuffic

Baseline 170, minimal- moderate variability

Stop pitocin

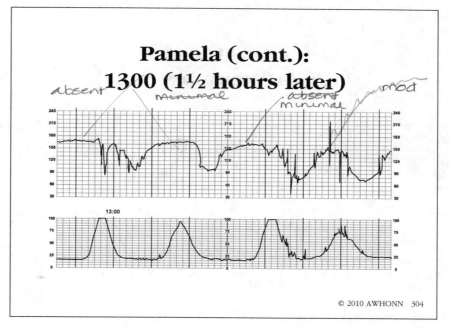

Stop pit

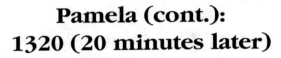

Pamela (cont.):
1320 (20 minutes later)

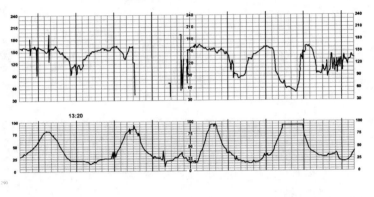

13:20

Pamela (cont.):
1340 (20 minutes later)

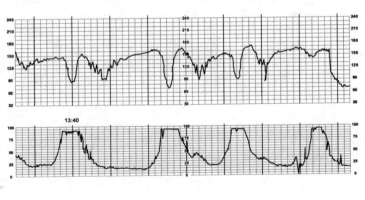

13:40

resting tone elevated.

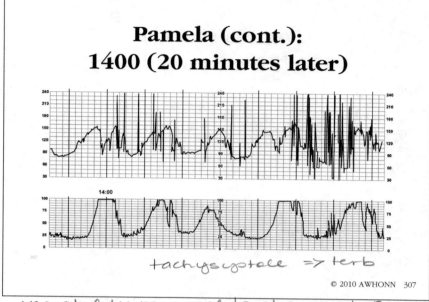

Pamela (cont.):
1400 (20 minutes later)

tachysystole => terb

© 2010 AWHONN 307

variability minimal to absent ∴ O₂
uterus not given opportunity to relax

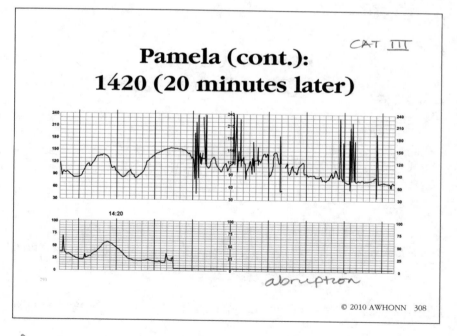

CAT III

Pamela (cont.):
1420 (20 minutes later)

abruption

© 2010 AWHONN 308

Baseline undeterminate, absent variability
recurrent variables

Pamela (cont.): Outcome

Neonatal outcome:

- 5 lb, 4 oz (2,381 g) male
- Apgar scores of 3/7/8 at 1, 5 and 10 minutes respectively
- Umbilical arterial cord blood gas values:
  - pH   7.0
  - pCO_2 125.0 mmHg
  - pO_2 12.4 mmHg
  - BD   22.6 mEq/L

© 2010 AWHONN 309

MIXED ACIDOSIS

Key Issues

- Respectful collaboration
- Comprehensive assessment, including patient input
- Critical decision making and reflection

© 2010 AWHONN 310

Key Issues (cont.)

- Physiologically based interventions
- Evolution of patterns over time
- Effective communication and documentation
- Taking action to resolve difficult situations

© 2010 AWHONN 311

Summary

- Clear goals
- Complete assessment
- Monitoring
- Core knowledge and skills

© 2010 AWHONN 312

The Collaborative Fetal Monitoring Process

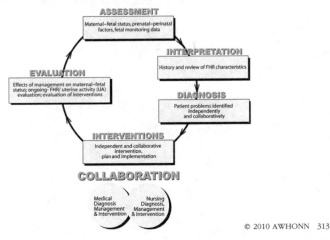

ASSESSMENT

Maternal–fetal status, prenatal–perinatal factors, fetal monitoring data

INTERPRETATION

History and review of FHR characteristics

EVALUATION

Effects of management on maternal–fetal status; ongoing- FHR/ uterine activity (UA) evaluation; evaluation of interventions

DIAGNOSIS

Patient problems identified independently and collaboratively

INTERVENTIONS

Independent and collaborative intervention, plan and implementation

COLLABORATION

Medical Diagnosis Management & Intervention

Nursing Diagnosis, Management & Intervention

© 2010 AWHONN   313

Plan

Do

Check

Act

Disclaimer: This course and all accompanying materials (publication) were developed by AWHONN in cooperation with PESG, as an educational resource for fetal heart monitoring. It presents general methods and techniques of practice that are currently acceptable, based on current research and used by recognized authorities. Proper care of individual patients may depend on many individual factors to be considered in clinical practice, as well as professional judgment in the techniques described herein. Clinical circumstances naturally vary, and professionals must use their own best judgment in accordance with the patients' needs and preferences, professional standards and institutional rules. Variations and innovations that are consistent with law, and that demonstrably improve the quality of patient care, should be encouraged.

AWHONN has sought to confirm the accuracy of the information presented herein and to describe generally accepted practices. However, AWHONN is not responsible for errors oromissions or for any consequences from application of the information in this resource and makes no warranty, expressed or implied, with respect to the contents of the publication.

Competent clinical practice depends on a broad array of personal characteristics, training, judgment, professional skills and institutional processes. This publication is simply one of many information resources. This publication is not intended to replace ongoing evaluation of knowledge and skills in the clinical setting. Nor has it been designed for use in hiring, promotion or termination decisions or in resolving legal disputes or issues of liability.

AWHONN believes that drug selection and dosage set forth in this text are in accordance with current recommendations and practice at the time of publication. However, in view of ongoing research, changes in government regulations, and the constant flow of information relating to drug therapy and drug reactions, the reader is urged to check other information available in other published sources for each drug for potential changes in indications, dosages and for added warnings and precautions. This is particularly important when the recommended agent is a new or infrequently employed drug.
   In addition, appropriate medication use may depend on unique factors such as individuals' health status, other medication use and other factors which the professional must consider in clinical practice.

© 2010 AWHONN   314

This workbook should be used to document answers for the skills stations and for Test B, if necessary.

Please retain this workbook for your records and do not send it to AWHONN or to the Professional Education Services Group.

Documentation Flowsheet

Date of Record: _____						
		TIME				
Cervix		Dilation				
		Effacement				
		Station				
Fetal Heart		Baseline Rate				
		Variability				
		Accelerations				
		Decelerations				
		STIM/pH				
		Monitor Mode				
Uterine Activity		Frequency				
		Duration				
		Intensity				
		Resting Tone				
		Monitor Mode				
		Coping				
		Pain				
		Maternal Position				
		O_2/LPM/Mask				
		IV				
Nurse Initials						

AWHONN FETAL HEART MONITORING PROGRAM

Skill Station: Integration of Fetal Heart Monitoring Knowledge and Practice

Practice Case Answer Sheet

CASE STUDY #_____

1. Variability:
    a. absent (undetectable) _____
    b. minimal (>0 but ≤5 bpm) _____
    c. moderate (6–25 bpm) _____
    d. marked (>25 bpm) _____
    e. unable to determine _____

2. Baseline FHR: _____

3. Contractions:
    Frequency _____
    Duration _____
    Intensity _____
    Resting Tonus _____

4. Accelerations and decelerations: When present, circle P if <u>periodic</u> and E if <u>episodic</u>.

Accelerations	P	E
Early decelerations	P	E
Variable decelerations	P	E
Late decelerations	P	E
Prolonged decelerations	P	E

5. List possible underlying physiologic mechanisms or rationales for observed patterns:

6. List actions and interventions indicated, based on overall interpretation (physiologic based, instrumentation based and further assessments):

AWHONN FETAL HEART MONITORING PROGRAM

Skill Station: Integration of Fetal Heart Monitoring Knowledge and Practice

Practice Case Answer Sheet

CASE STUDY #_____

1. Variability:
   a. absent (undetectable) _____
   b. minimal (>0 but ≤5 bpm) _____
   c. moderate (6–25 bpm) _____
   d. marked (>25 bpm) _____
   e. unable to determine _____

2. Baseline FHR: _____

3. Contractions:
   Frequency _____
   Duration _____
   Intensity _____
   Resting Tonus _____

4. Accelerations and decelerations: When present, circle P if _periodic_ and E if _episodic_.

Accelerations	P	E
Early decelerations	P	E
Variable decelerations	P	E
Late decelerations	P	E
Prolonged decelerations	P	E

5. List possible underlying physiologic mechanisms or rationales for observed patterns:

6. List actions and interventions indicated, based on overall interpretation (physiologic based, instrumentation based and further assessments):

AWHONN FETAL HEART MONITORING PROGRAM

Skill Station: Integration of Fetal Heart Monitoring Knowledge and Practice

Practice Case Answer Sheet

CASE STUDY #_____

1. Variability: a. absent (undetectable)   _____

b. minimal (>0 but ≤5 bpm)   _____

c. moderate (6–25 bpm)   _____

d. marked (>25 bpm)   _____

e. unable to determine   _____

2. Baseline FHR: _____

3. Contractions: Frequency   _____

Duration   _____

Intensity   _____

Resting Tonus   _____

4. Accelerations and decelerations: When present, circle P if <u>periodic</u> and E if <u>episodic</u>.

Accelerations   P   E
Early decelerations   P   E
Variable decelerations   P   E
Late decelerations   P   E
Prolonged decelerations P   E

5. List possible underlying physiologic mechanisms or rationales for observed patterns:

6. List actions and interventions indicated, based on overall interpretation (physiologic based, instrumentation based and further assessments):

AWHONN FETAL HEART MONITORING PROGRAM

Skill Station: Integration of Fetal Heart Monitoring Knowledge and Practice

Practice Case Answer Sheet

CASE STUDY #_____

1. Variability: a. absent (undetectable)   _____

         b. minimal (>0 but ≤5 bpm)   _____

         c. moderate (6–25 bpm)   _____

         d. marked (>25 bpm)   _____

         e. unable to determine   _____

2. Baseline FHR: _____

3. Contractions: Frequency   _____

         Duration   _____

         Intensity   _____

         Resting Tonus   _____

4. Accelerations and decelerations: When present, circle P if <u>periodic</u> and E if <u>episodic</u>.

    Accelerations   P   E
    Early decelerations   P   E
    Variable decelerations   P   E
    Late decelerations   P   E
    Prolonged decelerations   P   E

5. List possible underlying physiologic mechanisms or rationales for observed patterns:

6. List actions and interventions indicated, based on overall interpretation (physiologic based, instrumentation based and further assessments):

AWHONN FETAL HEART MONITORING PROGRAM

Skill Station: Integration of Fetal Heart Monitoring Knowledge and Practice

Practice Case Answer Sheet

CASE STUDY #_____

1. Variability:
   a. absent (undetectable) _____
   b. minimal (>0 but ≤5 bpm) _____
   c. moderate (6–25 bpm) _____
   d. marked (>25 bpm) _____
   e. unable to determine _____

2. Baseline FHR: _____

3. Contractions:
   Frequency _____
   Duration _____
   Intensity _____
   Resting Tonus _____

4. Accelerations and decelerations: When present, circle P if <u>periodic</u> and E if <u>episodic</u>.

Accelerations	P	E
Early decelerations	P	E
Variable decelerations	P	E
Late decelerations	P	E
Prolonged decelerations	P	E

5. List possible underlying physiologic mechanisms or rationales for observed patterns:

6. List actions and interventions indicated, based on overall interpretation (physiologic based, instrumentation based and further assessments):

AWHONN FETAL HEART MONITORING PROGRAM

Skill Station: Integration of Fetal Heart Monitoring Knowledge and Practice

Practice Case Answer Sheet

CASE STUDY #_____

1. Variability:
   a. absent (undetectable) _____
   b. minimal (>0 but ≤5 bpm) _____
   c. moderate (6–25 bpm) _____
   d. marked (>25 bpm) _____
   e. unable to determine _____

2. Baseline FHR: _____

3. Contractions:
   Frequency _____
   Duration _____
   Intensity _____
   Resting Tonus _____

4. Accelerations and decelerations: When present, circle P if <u>periodic</u> and E if <u>episodic</u>.

Accelerations	P	E
Early decelerations	P	E
Variable decelerations	P	E
Late decelerations	P	E
Prolonged decelerations	P	E

5. List possible underlying physiologic mechanisms or rationales for observed patterns:

6. List actions and interventions indicated, based on overall interpretation (physiologic based, instrumentation based and further assessments):

AWHONN FETAL HEART MONITORING PROGRAM

Skill Station: Integration of Fetal Heart Monitoring Knowledge and Practice

Practice Case Answer Sheet

CASE STUDY #_____

1. Variability: a. absent (undetectable)   _____

                       b. minimal (>0 but ≤5 bpm)   _____

                       c. moderate (6–25 bpm)   _____

                       d. marked (>25 bpm)   _____

                       e. unable to determine   _____

2. Baseline FHR: _____

3. Contractions: Frequency   _____

                      Duration   _____

                      Intensity   _____

                      Resting Tonus   _____

4. Accelerations and decelerations: When present, circle P if <u>periodic</u> and E if <u>episodic</u>.

Accelerations	P	E
Early decelerations	P	E
Variable decelerations	P	E
Late decelerations	P	E
Prolonged decelerations	P	E

5. List possible underlying physiologic mechanisms or rationales for observed patterns:

6. List actions and interventions indicated, based on overall interpretation (physiologic based, instrumentation based and further assessments):

AWHONN FETAL HEART MONITORING PROGRAM

Skill Station: Integration of Fetal Heart Monitoring Knowledge and Practice

Practice Case Answer Sheet

CASE STUDY #_____

1. Variability: a. absent (undetectable)   _____

                       b. minimal (>0 but ≤5 bpm)   _____

                       c. moderate (6–25 bpm)   _____

                       d. marked (>25 bpm)   _____

                       e. unable to determine   _____

2. Baseline FHR: _____

3. Contractions: Frequency   _____

                       Duration   _____

                       Intensity   _____

                       Resting Tonus   _____

4. Accelerations and decelerations: When present, circle P if <u>periodic</u> and E if <u>episodic</u>.

Accelerations	P	E
Early decelerations	P	E
Variable decelerations	P	E
Late decelerations	P	E
Prolonged decelerations	P	E

5. List possible underlying physiologic mechanisms or rationales for observed patterns:

6. List actions and interventions indicated, based on overall interpretation (physiologic based, instrumentation based and further assessments):

AWHONN FETAL HEART MONITORING PROGRAM

Skill Station: Integration of Fetal Heart Monitoring Knowledge and Practice

Practice Case Answer Sheet

CASE STUDY #_____

1. Variability:
    a. absent (undetectable)   _____
    b. minimal (>0 but ≤5 bpm)   _____
    c. moderate (6–25 bpm)   _____
    d. marked (>25 bpm)   _____
    e. unable to determine   _____

2. Baseline FHR: _____

3. Contractions:
    Frequency   _____
    Duration   _____
    Intensity   _____
    Resting Tonus   _____

4. Accelerations and decelerations: When present, circle P if _periodic_ and E if _episodic_.

Accelerations	P	E
Early decelerations	P	E
Variable decelerations	P	E
Late decelerations	P	E
Prolonged decelerations	P	E

5. List possible underlying physiologic mechanisms or rationales for observed patterns:

6. List actions and interventions indicated, based on overall interpretation (physiologic based, instrumentation based and further assessments):

AWHONN FETAL HEART MONITORING PROGRAM

Skill Station: Integration of Fetal Heart Monitoring Knowledge and Practice

Practice Case Answer Sheet

CASE STUDY #_____

1. Variability:
   a. absent (undetectable) _____
   b. minimal (>0 but ≤5 bpm) _____
   c. moderate (6–25 bpm) _____
   d. marked (>25 bpm) _____
   e. unable to determine _____

2. Baseline FHR: _____

3. Contractions:
   Frequency _____
   Duration _____
   Intensity _____
   Resting Tonus _____

4. Accelerations and decelerations: When present, circle P if <u>periodic</u> and E if <u>episodic</u>.

Accelerations	P	E
Early decelerations	P	E
Variable decelerations	P	E
Late decelerations	P	E
Prolonged decelerations	P	E

5. List possible underlying physiologic mechanisms or rationales for observed patterns:

6. List actions and interventions indicated, based on overall interpretation (physiologic based, instrumentation based and further assessments):

AWHONN FETAL HEART MONITORING PROGRAM

Skill Station: Integration of Fetal Heart Monitoring Knowledge and Practice

Practice Case Answer Sheet

CASE STUDY #_____

1. Variability: a. absent (undetectable)   _____

                     b. minimal (>0 but ≤5 bpm)   _____

                     c. moderate (6–25 bpm)   _____

                     d. marked (>25 bpm)   _____

                     e. unable to determine   _____

2. Baseline FHR: _____

3. Contractions: Frequency   _____

                     Duration   _____

                     Intensity   _____

                     Resting Tonus   _____

4. Accelerations and decelerations: When present, circle P if <u>periodic</u> and E if <u>episodic</u>.

Accelerations	P	E
Early decelerations	P	E
Variable decelerations	P	E
Late decelerations	P	E
Prolonged decelerations	P	E

5. List possible underlying physiologic mechanisms or rationales for observed patterns:

6. List actions and interventions indicated, based on overall interpretation (physiologic based, instrumentation based and further assessments):

SKILL STATION: COMMUNICATION OF FETAL HEART MONITORING DATA PRACTICE

Practice Exercise I

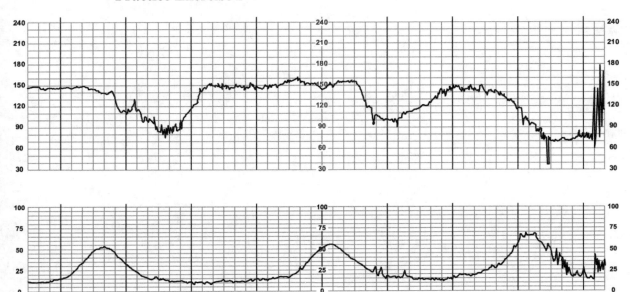

a) Please document your interpretation of this tracing:
   a. Baseline rate   _____
   b. Variability   _____
   c. Accelerations   _____
   d. Decelerations   _____
   e. Uterine activity _____

b) Be prepared to discuss what you would report to another provider about this tracing.

Practice Exercise I
Correct Responses

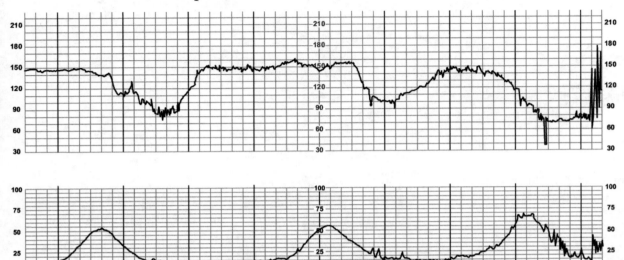

c) Please document your interpretation of this tracing:
   a. Baseline rate   150 bpm
   b. Variability   minimal
   c. Accelerations   none
   d. Decelerations   late and variable
   e. Uterine activity   every 2½–3 minutes & 70–90 seconds duration

d) Components of the description of what you would report to another provider about this tracing include:

   "The FHR baseline is 150 bpm with minimal variability and recurrent late and periodic variable decelerations. The tracing requires your immediate bedside evaluation. When can I expect that you will be here?"

Practice Exercise II

Please document your interpretation of the tracing below on the flowsheet provided. The tracing is obtained using a spiral electrode and intrauterine pressure catheter.

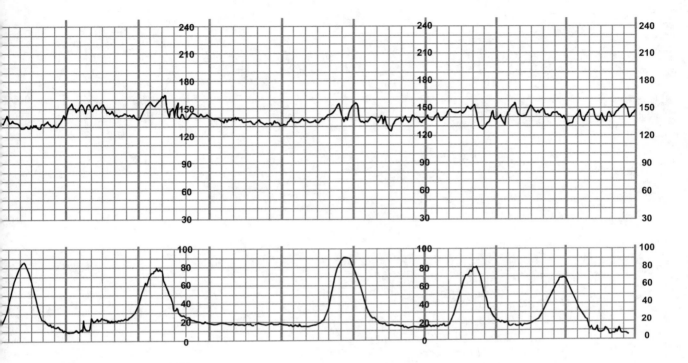

Practice Exercise II—Documentation Flowsheet

Date of Record: _____

	TIME				
Cervix	Dilation				
	Effacement				
	Station				
Fetal Heart	Baseline Rate				
	Variability				
	Accelerations				
	Decelerations				
	STIM/pH				
	Monitor Mode				
Uterine Activity	Frequency				
	Duration				
	Intensity				
	Resting Tone				
	Monitor Mode				
	Coping				
	Maternal Position				
	O_2/LPM/Mask				
	IV				
Nurse Initials					

Practice Exercise II—Correct Documentation

Date of Record: _____					
	TIME				
Cervix	Dilation				
	Effacement				
	Station				
Fetal Heart	Variability	moderate			
	Baseline Rate	140			
	Accelerations	present			
	Decelerations	Ø			
	STIM/pH				
	Monitor Mode	FSE			
Uterine Activity	Frequency	1–3			
	Duration	40–50			
	Intensity	70–90			
	Resting Tone	10–15			
	Monitor Mode	IUPC			
	Coping				
	Maternal Position				
	O_2/LPM/Mask				
	IV				
Nurse Initials					

SKILL STATION: COMMUNICATION OF FETAL HEART MONITORING DATA TEST

NOTE: There are two separate exercises in the testing component of this station. Please do both of them.

Exercise I (See the tracings and flowsheet on the following page.)

Monica is a G_3, P_2 admitted in early labor at 39 weeks' gestation. No risk factors are noted, and no antepartum testing was done. She had two previous low-risk pregnancies; these children are ages 8 and 10 years old. Her vaginal exam reveals 3 cm, 90% effaced, floating and cephalic presentation. Membranes are intact. US and toco monitors are in place.

Instructions

A. Interpret the monitor tracings on the next page and document your findings in two separate columns on the flowsheet provided. Please include any additional troubleshooting or interventions you would provide in the appropriate spaces in the flowsheet.

B. Assume that after the second monitor tracing at 15:30 you phone in report to the physician, describing the observed pattern. You are told to call again in one hour if there is no change. Document your short verbal response to the physician in the space below and also describe the next clinical action you will take in response to the physician's order. Take the scenario as far as you believe is appropriate.

_____

_____

_____

_____

_____

Exercise I
US, TOCO

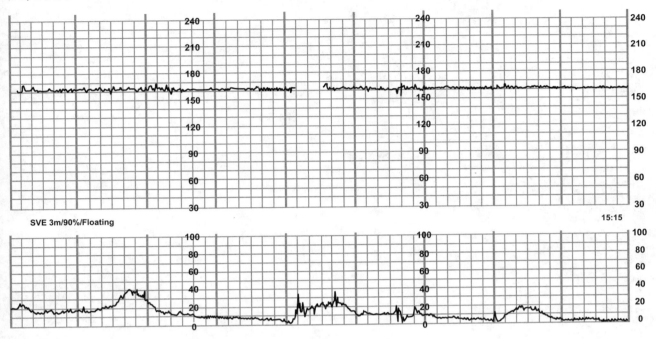

SVE 3m/90%/Floating

15:15

Exercise II (continued)
SE, TOCO

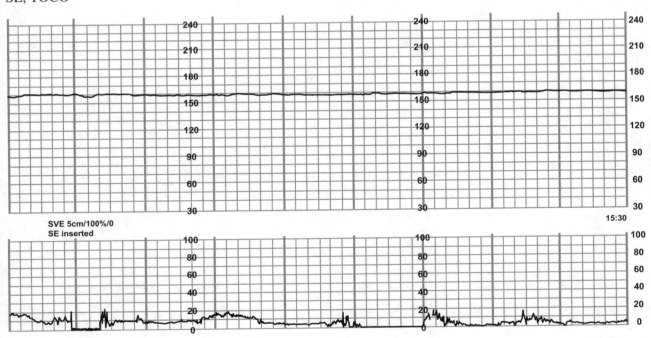

SVE 5cm/100%/0
SE inserted

15:30

Documentation Flowsheet

		TIME				
Cervix	Dilation					
	Effacement					
	Station					
Fetal Heart	Baseline Rate					
	Variability					
	Accelerations					
	Decelerations					
	STIM/pH					
	Monitor Mode					
Uterine Activity	Frequency					
	Duration					
	Intensity					
	Resting Tone					
	Monitor Mode					
	Coping					
	Pain					
	Maternal Position					
	O_2/LPM/Mask					
	IV					
	Nurse Initials					

Date of Record: _____

Exercise I
Documentation Flowsheet

Date of Record: _____					
	TIME				
Cervix	Dilation				
	Effacement				
	Station				
Fetal Heart	Baseline Rate				
	Variability				
	Accelerations				
	Decelerations				
	STIM/pH				
	Monitor Mode				
Uterine Activity	Frequency				
	Duration				
	Intensity				
	Resting Tone				
	Monitor Mode				
	Coping				
	Pain				
	Maternal Position				
	O_2/LPM/Mask				
	IV				
Nurse Initials					

NOTE: There are two separate exercises on this test. Please do both of them.

Exercise II

For this exercise you will watch a scenario depicting nurse-to-nurse reporting. This scenario can be viewed more than once if needed. The objective of the testing component of the DVD is that you will document four omissions you noted in the nurse-to-nurse report. There are more than four omissions in the scenario, but you are only required to list four.

1. _____
2. _____
3. _____
4. _____

SKILL STATION: COMMUNICATION SCENARIO CRITIQUE WORKSHEET

Please use this page to list your answers for the critique of communication about fetal heart monitoring information (you may write on the back of the page if needed).

Nurse-to-Nurse Report
Data included in the report:

_____

_____

_____

_____

_____

_____

_____

_____

Nurse-to-Nurse Report
Data omitted from the report:

_____

_____

_____

_____

_____

_____

_____

_____

Nurse-to-Patient Education
Data included in the education:

_____

_____

_____

_____

_____

_____

Nurse-to-Patient Education
Data that may have been added:

_____

_____

_____

_____

_____

_____

Nurse-to-Physician Report
Data included in the report:

_____

_____

_____

_____

_____

_____

_____

_____

Nurse-to-Physician Report
Data omitted from the report:

_____

_____

_____

_____

_____

_____

_____

_____

Nurse-to-Patient Education
Data included in the education:

_____
_____
_____
_____
_____
_____

Nurse-to-Physician Report
Data included in the report:

_____
_____
_____
_____
_____
_____
_____
_____
_____
_____
_____
_____

Nurse-to-Charge Nurse Report
Data included in the report:

_____
_____
_____
_____
_____
_____
_____
_____
_____
_____

Nurse-to-Patient Education
Data that may have been added:

_____
_____
_____
_____
_____
_____

Nurse-to-Physician Report
Data omitted from the report:

_____
_____
_____
_____
_____
_____
_____
_____
_____
_____
_____
_____

Nurse-to-Charge Nurse Report
Data omitted from the report:

_____
_____
_____
_____
_____
_____
_____
_____
_____
_____

Charge Nurse-to-Nurse Manager Report
Data included in the report:

_____
_____
_____
_____
_____
_____
_____
_____

Charge Nurse-to-Manager Report
Data omitted from the report:

_____
_____
_____
_____
_____
_____
_____
_____

INTERMEDIATE FETAL MONITORING COURSE
TEST B ANSWER SHEET

Participant Name: _____

Course No: _____

Date: _____

Test B is to be administered only if the participant does not successfully complete Test A. If the participant successfully completes Test B, Competence Validation will be awarded. If the participant fails both Test A and Test B, Competence Validation should not be awarded.

The corresponding original questions should be retained by the instructor.
This form should not be mailed back to the AWHONN processing center.

Answer Sheet

	A	B	C		A	B	C		A	B	C		A	B	C		A	B	C
1	○	○	○	11	○	○	○	21	○	○	○	31	○	○	○	41	○	○	○
2	○	○	○	12	○	○	○	22	○	○	○	32	○	○	○	42	○	○	○
3	○	○	○	13	○	○	○	23	○	○	○	33	○	○	○	43	○	○	○
4	○	○	○	14	○	○	○	24	○	○	○	34	○	○	○	44	○	○	○
5	○	○	○	15	○	○	○	25	○	○	○	35	○	○	○	45	○	○	○
6	○	○	○	16	○	○	○	26	○	○	○	36	○	○	○	46	○	○	○
7	○	○	○	17	○	○	○	27	○	○	○	37	○	○	○	47	○	○	○
8	○	○	○	18	○	○	○	28	○	○	○	38	○	○	○	48	○	○	○
9	○	○	○	19	○	○	○	29	○	○	○	39	○	○	○	49	○	○	○
10	○	○	○	20	○	○	○	30	○	○	○	40	○	○	○	50	○	○	○